Praise for *A Straight Talking Introduction to Th[illegible]py*

So much is written for therapists [illegible] upport clients with a range of probl[illegible] ho are the clients and are wo[illegible] eutic 'process'. Indeed, the [illegible] rent types of therapies and t[illegible] ne available are sometimes [illegible] that, in plain and accessible la[illegible] ole endeavour – from start to finish. In w[illegible] rful book, Wotton and Johnston have created an i[illegible] c resource for anyone thinking of therapy, to best position them to walk through the door (or log in online) with more confidence and understanding of what might happen. This compelling and highly readable book might be seen as the first part of therapy itself, in equipping the client with insight, knowledge and autonomy as they take their first steps.
Andrew Reeves, Professor in Counselling Professions and Mental Health, University of Chester

This is a well-researched and useful resource, especially for those who don't qualify or can't wait for NHS help and who need to access services from the voluntary sector or from private providers. It's the kind of book I'd recommend professionally and personally.
Claire Vilarrubi, forensic psychologist

Given how life-changingly important therapy can be and how mind-bogglingly confusing the world of therapy is, it's a wonder we don't have more books like this. Drawing on their deep commitment to therapy's potential, Wotton and Johnston offer a text that is as accessible and jargon-free as it is comprehensive and solidly researched. From choosing best therapist for your needs, understanding all your options, staying safe, and getting the most out of what might be one of the most important decisions of your life, this book has it all. Wonderfully comprehensive and well written, this is a must-read for anyone considering therapy.
Dr Aaron Balick, PhD, psychotherapist and author

Matt Wotton and Graham Johnston are therapists on a mission to explain the world of the mind and how therapy can help many of us live more satisfying lives. Avoiding jargon, this short book accurately explains what talking therapy is like and can achieve, as well as highlighting relevant research. The authors are encouraging and supportive, but also honest about the hard work that therapy may require. I sense that their inclusive, readable style will convert many readers to take the plunge and look for a therapist of their own.
Louise Chunn, founder of therapist-matching platform Welldoing

Knowing where to start when you think you might need help from a therapist is a daunting prospect. You don't know what you don't know. This book is a must – a credible, straightforward and objective guide to the world of therapy. It's well researched, clearly written, easy to read and understand.
Jeremy Lowe, Investment Manager at a Top 20 Hedge Fund

As every GP knows, referring a patient for therapy often involves a long wait and very little choice in the treatment they get. And sometimes patients just can't wait. Those lucky enough to be able to find low cost therapy or pay for therapy themselves need this book to help them navigate the minefield of unregulated private practice. It tells you what to look for and, just as importantly, what to avoid. It's exactly the kind of book I would have recommended to my patients.
Dr Ivor Robinson, retired GP

A STRAIGHT TALKING INTRODUCTION TO

THERAPY

WHAT IT IS, WHY IT WORKS, HOW TO GET IT

MATT WOTTON &
GRAHAM JOHNSTON

PCCS BOOKS

First published 2023

PCCS Books Ltd
Wyastone Business Park
Wyastone Leys
Monmouth
NP25 3SR
UK

Tel +44 (0)1600 891509
contact@pccs-books.co.uk
www.pccs-books.co.uk

A Straight Talking Introduction to Therapy: What it is, why it works, how to get it

British Library Cataloguing in Publication Data.
A catalogue record for this book is available from the British Library

ISBNs
paperback – 978 1 915220 33 2
epub – 978 1 915220 34 9

Cover design by Jason Anscomb
Printed in the UK by Severnprint, Gloucester

A Straight Talking Introduction to Therapy: What it is, why it works, how to get it

Contents

Dedications

To all the people who I've loved and let down. But mostly to Fern.
(MW)

To my parents. I always felt loved. That's more than good enough.
(GJ)

About the authors

Matt Wotton and Graham Johnston worked for two decades at the centre of government on some of the most complex problems facing the country, shaping decisions that affected millions of people. In the last decade, they left government, retrained as psychotherapists and set up the London Centre for Applied Psychology, which provides evidence-based training to mental health professionals and consults to business on mental health and wellbeing at work.

Matt is a former Chair of the Bowlby Centre. He has been a member of the Prison and Probation Board, studied at the London Business School and has an MBA from Warwick University. He contributes to the national press on relationship breakdown, managing mental health in sports, and how therapy and psychological coaching impact high performance.

Graham was Director of Policy at the Bowlby Centre. He has studied in the US and has an MBA from Imperial College, London. He writes and speaks on relationships and parenting in the 21st century, the challenges of midlife, and how therapy sits alongside developments in technology, AI, psychedelics and psychiatric medication.

Acknowledgements

We would like to thank our editor at PCCS Books, Catherine Jackson. She's been just lovely throughout. Tough on adjectives and Oxford commas; fair on the evidence and on us.

We'd also like to thank Charles, who encouraged us to get on and write the book, and then put his money where his mouth is.

This book wouldn't seem to have much to do with how the UK government operates – but that's where we learned our trade: sifting and weighing evidence fairly to give clear, unbiased advice. We don't miss those days much, to be honest, but we do wish our old friends and colleagues well.

Outside of all things therapy, we want to thank our friends, who don't take us or our insights too seriously and who remind us that there are lots of ways to stay healthy and that life is for living.

Matt: I would especially like to thank Gita, who suffered through the early drafts, had date nights taken up with mental health chat, and did even more of the heavy lifting at home. She's the best wife ever. I'd also like to thank the best boys ever – Patrick and Hari. We finally have a real book 'like what you can get in libraries'; now let's get back to playing football and FIFA. Also Dom, who I run everything by. If there is anything in this book you disagree with or don't like, it's because I didn't run that part past him. And finally, Graham 'we're not wasting our time writing a book' Johnston, my co-author, business partner and friend – it's been a real pleasure.

Graham: The biggest thanks to my home team – Helen, who stood by my side when times were very dark and gave me the reason to want to emerge out the other side; Grace, Freya and Ezra, who run me ragged but offer me a glimpse into something divine on a daily basis. Thanks to Tom and Paul for the beers, the chats and the laughs, especially in some of those dark times. Thanks to my clients, old and new: it's a privilege to spend my working life with you. Finally, I'd like to thank Matt, who convinced me it was worth the time and effort required to write a book. He made it a lot easier and more fun than I thought it would be. Thanks, mate.

Introducing the *Straight Talking Introductions* series

What are mental health problems?

Much of what is written and spoken about emotional distress or mental health problems implies that they are illnesses. This can lead us all too easily to believe that we no longer have to think about mental health problems, because illness is best left to doctors. They are the illness experts, and psychiatrists are the doctors who specialise in mental illness. This series of books is different because we don't think that all mental health problems should automatically be regarded as illnesses.

If mental health problems aren't necessarily illnesses, it means that the burden of responsibility for distress in our lives should not be shouldered entirely by doctors and psychiatrists. All citizens have a responsibility, however small, in creating a world where everyone has a decent opportunity to live a fulfilling life. This is a contentious idea, but one that we want to advance, alongside the dominant medical view.

Rather than accept that the ways of understanding and solutions to mental health problems are 'owned' by the medical profession, we will take a good look at alternatives that involve the users of psychiatric services, their carers, families, friends and other 'ordinary people' taking control of their own lives, and that means all of us. One of the tools required in order to become active in mental health issues, whether your own or other people's, is knowledge. This series of books is a starting point for anyone who wants to know more about mental health.

How these books are written

Information

We want these books to be understandable, so we use everyday language wherever possible. The books could have been almost completely jargon-free, but we thought that including some technical and medical terms would be helpful. Most doctors, psychiatrists and psychologists use the medical model of mental illness and manuals to help them diagnose mental health problems. The medical model and the diagnostic manuals use a particular set of terms to describe what doctors think of as 'conditions'. Although these words aren't very good at describing individual people's experiences, they are used a lot in psychiatric and psychological services, so we thought it would be helpful to define these terms as we went along and use them in a way that might help readers understand what the professionals mean. We don't expect that psychiatrists and psychologists and others working in mental health services will stop using medical terminology (although we think it would be respectful for them to drop it when talking to their patients and their families), so these books should help you get used to and learn *their* language.

The books also contain resources for further learning. As well as lists of books, websites and organisations at the end of the book, there are references. These will not be important to everyone, but they do tell the reader where information – a claim about effectiveness, an argument for or against, or a quotation – has come from, so you can follow it up if you wish.

Being realistic and reassuring

Our aim is to be realistic – neither overly optimistic nor pessimistic. Things are nearly always more complicated than we would like them to be. Honest evaluations of mental health problems, of what might cause them, of what can help and of what the likely outcome might be are, like so much in life, somewhere in between. For the vast majority of people, it would be wrong to say that they have an illness from which they will never recover. But it would be equally wrong to say that they will be completely unchanged by the distressing thoughts and feelings they are having. Life is an accumulation of experiences. There is almost certainly no pill, or any other treatment for that matter, that will take us back to 'how we were before'. There are many things we can do (and we look at lots of them in this series), in collaboration with doctors, psychiatrists, psychologists and counsellors, and, indeed, everyone working in mental health services, with the help of our friends and family, or on our own, that stand a good chance of helping us feel better and build a constructive life, with hope for the future.

Of course, we understand that the experiences dealt with in these books can sometimes be so overwhelming, confusing and terrifying that people will try to escape from them by withdrawing, going mad or even trying to kill themselves. This happens when our usual coping strategies fail us. We accept that killing oneself is, in some circumstances, a rational act – that, for the person in question, it can make a lot of sense. Nonetheless, we believe that much of the distress that underpins such an extreme course of action, from which there can be no turning back, is avoidable. For this reason, all of the books in this series point towards realistic hope and recovery.

Debates

There is no single convenient answer to many of the most important questions explored in these books. No matter how badly we might wish for a simple answer, what we have is a series of debates – or arguments, more like – between stakeholders, and there are many stakeholders whose voices demand space in these books. We use the word 'stakeholders' here because service users, carers, friends, family, doctors, psychologists, psychiatrists, nurses and other healthcare workers, scientists in drug companies, therapists and, indeed, all citizens have a stake in how our society understands and deals with problems of mental health. It is simultaneously big business and intimately personal, and many things in between. As we go along, we try to explain how someone's stake in distress (including our own, where we can see it), whether professional or personal, can influence their experience and judgement.

While we want to present competing (sometimes opposing) viewpoints, we don't want to leave the reader high and dry to evaluate complicated debates on their own. We will try to present reasonable conclusions that might point in certain directions for personal action. Above all, though, we believe that knowledge is power and that the better informed you are, even though the information might be conflicting, the more able you will be to make sound decisions.

It's also useful to be reminded that the professionals involved in helping distressed people are themselves caught in the same flow of conflicting information. It is their *job*, however, to interpret it in our service, so that the best solutions are available to as many people as possible. You may have noticed that the word 'best' brings with it certain challenges, not least defining what we mean when we use this term. Perhaps 'the best' means the most effective? However, even using words like 'effective' doesn't completely clear up the puzzle. An effective treatment for an employer could be the one that returns a member of staff to work quickly; for a parent, it could be one that makes their child feel happier and calmer. For the government or the NHS, or someone running a private healthcare business, 'effective' might mean 'cost-effective'. This brings us to evidence.

Evidence

Throughout these books there will be material that we will present as 'evidence'. This is one of the most contentious terms to be found in this series. One person's evidence is another person's fanciful mythology and yet another person's oppressive propaganda. Nevertheless, the term crops up increasingly in everyday settings, most relevantly when we hear of 'evidence-based practice'. The idea behind this term is that the treatments psychologists and psychiatrists offer should be those that 'work'. Crudely put, there should be some evidence that, say, talking about problems or taking a prescribed drug actually helps people feel better. We encounter a real problem, however, when trying to evaluate this evidence, as the books in this series will demonstrate. We will try not to discount any 'evidence' out of hand, but we will critically evaluate it, and we will do this with a bias towards scientific evaluation.

The types of evidence that will be covered in these books, along with their positive and negative points, include the following.

Research methods, numbers and statistics

On the one hand, the logic of most research is simple, but on the other hand, the way things have to be arranged to avoid bias in the results can lead to a perplexing system of measurements. Even the experts lose the sense of it, sometimes. We'll try to explain the logic of studies, but almost certainly leave out the details. You can look these up yourself if you wish.

The books in this series look at research into a wide range of issues relating to mental health problems, including the experience of distress, what is known about the causes of problems, and their prevention and treatment. Different research methods are appropriate for each of these areas, so we will be looking at different types of research as we go along. We say this now because many readers may be most familiar with studies into the *effective treatments* of distress, and we want to emphasise that there are many other credible and valid sources of essential information about distress that are sometimes overlooked.

You may have come across the idea that some research methods are 'better' than others – that they constitute a 'gold standard'. In the case of research into the effectiveness of different treatments, the gold standard is usually considered to be randomised controlled trials (RCTs). In simple terms, RCTs are complex (and often very expensive) experiments in which a group of individuals who all suffer from the same problem are allocated randomly to a treatment (such as a drug or a form of talking therapy) or a 'control' treatment (at its simplest, no treatment at all, or a dummy pill or 'placebo') to test if the treatment works. We are not necessarily convinced that RCTs always *are* the best way of proving the effectiveness of different treatments, but they are, currently, the method given most credence by the bodies that control funding and what it is spent on, such as (in England) the National Institute for Health and Care Excellence (NICE) – so we need to understand them.

Before it is accepted by academics and clinicians, research must be written up and published in a journal that asks independent people to read it, to make sure that it is *bona fide* and that no glaring mistakes have been made. In recent years, a number of high-profile academics and scientific commentators have drawn attention to possible problems with this system of quality control. This series of books is not the place to deal with these arguments, but where they impinge on the evidence in a particular area, we will make sure it is highlighted.

Personal experience

Personal experience is an important source of evidence, to the extent that, nowadays, people who have suffered debilitating psychiatric distress are sometimes called 'experts by experience'. Personal stories provide an essential counterbalance to the impersonal numbers and statistics often found in research projects such as RCTs. While not everyone is average, by definition most people are. Balancing the average results obtained from RCTs with some personal stories helps complete the picture and is now widely accepted, to the extent that it has given birth to the new field of 'survivor research'.

Understanding contexts

Widening our view to include people's families and lives and the cultural, economic, social and political settings in which we live completes the picture. Mental health problems are connected to the conditions in which we all live, just as much as they are connected to our biology. From the start, we want readers to know that, if there is one message or model that these books are trying to get across, it is that problems in mental health are more often than not the result of complex events in the environments in which we live and our reactions to them. These reactions can also be influenced by our biology and the way we have learned to think and feel. Hopefully, these books will help disentangle the puzzle of distress and provide positive suggestions and hope for us all, whether we work in the system, currently have mental health problems ourselves or are caring for or friends with someone who has.

We hope that readers of these books will feel empowered by what they learn and thereby feel more able to get the best out of mental health services. It would be wonderful if our efforts, directly or indirectly, influence the development of services that effectively address the emotional, social and practical needs of people with mental health problems.

Richard Bentall
Pete Sanders
2021

Introduction
Why we wrote this book

Good therapy can change your life. That's why we wrote this book.

We know this because we both work as psychotherapists and we see the changes in our clients. They stop worrying so much; they start making better decisions; they are kinder to themselves and the people around them; they take control of their careers and achieve more; they control their anger; they stop overeating; they are able to leave the house and exercise; they get on better with their boss or partner or children; they stand up for themselves; they start dating again.

In short, they take the necessary action to live fuller, richer lives. Of course, things still go wrong for them. Of course, life doesn't always work out for them. But they can cope. They can put setbacks into perspective, savour what they've got, express gratitude for the good things, move on and try again.

Don't just take our word for it. This is what the research shows too. Therapy works. For decades, research by some of the leading academics in this area (Lemma et al., 2011) has consistently shown that psychotherapy is effective, with an effect size larger than almost all interventions in cardiology and greater than the success rate of flu vaccinations (Wampold & Imel, 2015). Pause on that fact for a moment. The average effect size from those studies tells us that three-quarters of people who have therapy end up with better mental health than those who don't. That's 75 people in every 100. Although there is still debate about exactly what kind of therapy works best, there is almost no serious disagreement about its efficacy as a cost-effective way of relieving emotional distress

(Layard & Clark, 2015a), even when compared against medication or other medical treatments (Cuijpers et al., 2013, 2020; Lambert, 2013).

Therapy worked for us and it can work for you

We also know that therapy works because of personal experience – it made a difference in our own lives. It changed each of us dramatically for the better. For one of us, that was coming to terms with a short temper and the destruction it caused in relationships. Therapy was a way to understand and accept the reality of a compulsive and addictive personality that, if unchecked, could lead to some dark places.

Therapy meant the difference between being overwhelmed by emotions and working out ways to slow down, understand what was causing those feelings, weigh the cost of impulsive actions and make better decisions. Not perfectly. Not instantly. There were still people who got hurt along the way – and this book is dedicated to them. But things got better.

Those changes can be seen in the ability to form stable, long-term, harmonious relationships in a way that was impossible for many years. Without claiming to have reached anything near perfection, the difference between now and first entering therapy is the difference between night and day.

For the other one of us, it was recovery from a deep depression brought on by an all-consuming need to please others. That was combined with a perfectionism that could sometimes be helpful at work. It also meant being well liked. After all, who doesn't like someone who is focused on pleasing them, making them happy or making sure they feel important and valued as friends and partners? But, more often than not, it meant hitting a wall time and again, each time disappointment and imperfections reared their ugly heads. It meant being in a series of bad relationships where their own needs were ignored in favour of the other, in a desperate attempt to maintain stability and continue to be the 'good guy'.

Working with a good therapist meant learning to find ways to assert healthy boundaries, even when that meant disappointing others. It meant learning skills to tolerate the distress others felt without the need to rescue them. In short, it meant learning to be an imperfect adult, just like everyone else. Yes, there are still darker days, but the setbacks are shorter, relationships are stronger and feelings are expressed more honestly.

That's why, decades after those first experiences in therapy, we each gave up successful careers to retrain as psychotherapists. We both turned our backs on seemingly important, well-paid jobs, much to the surprise of colleagues and others. In the year before we retrained, one of us oversaw an international review for the then prime minister, travelling between New York, Washington, Sydney and Paris. The other was a chief of staff in a major government agency. But nothing compares with the pleasure of seeing someone make a change for the better in their life via therapy. When a person realises what is holding them back and they find a way to do something about that, it gives a feeling of satisfaction like no other. Therapy may not have the glamour of drinks on the lawn of the British Embassy in Washington D.C., but it's ultimately more satisfying and, in our opinion at least, more important.

Our experiences of therapy are not unique. Most people who've had therapy say that the experience helped them. BACP, the largest professional body of therapists in the UK, says that therapy and counselling 'change lives' (BACP, 2019). And 76% of people polled in a YouGov survey agree: more than three-quarters of people who had therapy said they would recommend it to a friend or family member (BACP, 2019). When you consider that those same people are spending considerable amounts of time and money and often talking about the darkest and most difficult aspects of their lives, that's a pretty high satisfaction rate.

One of the most influential psychologists of the 20th century, Martin Seligman (1995), cites research showing even higher rates of satisfaction in the US, where more than 90% of people who had therapy said they felt better by the end of it. There are some methodological flaws with surveys of this kind, but they are asking real people how they felt about real problems after working with real therapists. And what these people say overwhelmingly is that it was a helpful experience.

And that is why we set up the London Centre for Applied Psychology. We wanted to help other mental health professionals draw on the most effective treatments and deliver them in the most effective ways to the greatest number of people.

Mental health is (arguably) Britain's biggest social problem

This book is a logical extension of that. We now want to help the thousands of people in the UK each year who look for therapy to get the help and support they need. Therapy has never been more important in public life and mental health is now probably the UK's biggest social problem (Layard, 2005). Not convinced? Just consider these statistics.

A third of us are expected to experience a diagnosed mental illness at some point in our life (Layard & Clark, 2015b). One in four of us in England will experience a mental health problem of some kind each year, and one in six report experiencing a common mental health problem in any given week (Mind, 2020).

In developed countries, the World Health Organization (WHO) estimates that mental health problems account for nearly 40% of all illness, while stroke, cancer, heart disease, lung disease and diabetes together account for less than 20% (WHO, 2022). By 2030, WHO estimates that depression will be the biggest threat to public health worldwide (WHO, 2022). As many people die from suicide as from homicide and warfare combined, worldwide, and in the US, more people end their own life than are killed in road accidents (Centers for Disease Control and Prevention, 2013). In the UK, mental health problems give rise to nearly half of all absences from work through sickness (Health & Safety Executive, 2022). In short, the scale of mental ill health is mind boggling (Layard & Clark, 2015a).

Mental distress is painful enough, but increasingly its effects on physical health are seen and quantified too. In one study (Patten et al., 2008), people with depression were at least 50% more likely to develop heart disease, stroke, lung disease, asthma or arthritis. Problems with mental health also account for nearly half of the people claiming disability benefit (Cribb et al., 2022), and 40% of GP appointments now involve a mental health issue (Mind, 2018). Yet spending on mental health has failed to keep up with that need. Eleven major economies in the world have just one psychologist per 10,000 people, at most (Organisation for Economic Co-operation and Development, 2021). That's why so many people are left trying to manage their own mental health problems.

Most people who go to therapy are not 'mentally ill'

While severe depression and anxiety seem like obvious mental health issues, they are by no means the only problems for which people seek therapy. Mental health exists on a spectrum from feeling fine to feeling like you want to end it all. In between are all sorts of problems, ranging from feeling stuck, lonely or overwhelmed to experiencing episodes of panic, overeating or being deeply troubled by intrusive thoughts. Whether or not those problems are regarded and described as 'mental illness' depends on their frequency and severity (Foulkes, 2021), but many can be thought of as ordinary or 'normal' (Frances, 2013). And they are exactly the kinds of issues that millions of people seek help for every year, without crossing the threshold for psychiatric assessment or treatment.

For decades, dissenting voices have argued that the term 'mental illness' is an unhelpful label (see, for example, Szasz, 1961; Johnstone, 2021; Johnstone & Boyle et al., 2018). And there are good reasons for wanting to drop the notion of 'mental disorder' (Watson, 2019) and put the person first (Sanders & Tolan, 2023), rather than their supposed 'illness'. What is so 'disordered' about their feelings? Why do we assume they need 'treatment' to return them to some arbitrary notion of 'normal'?

But there is also a strong argument on the other side that some psychological experiences are so distressing and disabling that the labels of illness and disorder are not only useful but also necessary (Foulkes, 2021). They can be essential 'passports' to better help and more effective treatment, especially within the NHS.

In the end, as has been well said elsewhere (Filer, 2019), there is no uncontroversial way of talking about mental illness, including the phrase 'mental illness' itself. Some people prefer to think of their distress as similar to a physical illness and to consider themselves as a patient who needs medical treatment and looking after. A psychological diagnosis means being seen, believed and offered practical as well as medical help. But for others, it brings stigma, and medications with unwelcome side effects.

Wherever you are positioned on the issue, it's worth knowing that, right from the very early days of therapy, the majority of those who sought it came seeking personal growth, support and guidance during difficult times, not because they were ill (Elkins,

2009). Many say the same today (Elkins, 2009). Therapy exists not just to treat so-called mental illness; it is also now the most accepted way for people to seek support for personal development or get help and guidance in times of distress and personal difficulties (Bellah et al., 2007). This is particularly so as society has become more individualistic, with fewer forms of traditional support and guidance (Putnam, 1995).

All of which means that therapy, in all its guises – whether for profound mental distress, for everyday problems or for personal and professional development – is booming. A recent YouGov poll showed that 85% of people now think that it's a good idea to seek therapy for a problem before it gets out of hand, and almost three-quarters agree that people might be happier if they talked to a therapist (BACP, 2019). The UK has moved a long way from the stiff upper lip caricature.

If we combine the number of people who experience common mental health problems with those seeking help for everyday problems or looking for personal development, that's a lot of people now going to therapy. And even more are thinking about doing so. If you're one of them, then you need to know how to get the very best help possible.

Too often, people get bad therapy

It's important to emphasise here that we are writing about individual therapy for adults, not about children's therapy or therapy for couples (although many of the same principles will apply). We are also writing about therapy provided by qualified practitioners either in a public health service (the NHS, so free at point of delivery), in the voluntary sector (sometimes free and often at a reduced rate) or in private practice (the client pays). Most of the 75,000 and counting qualified, registered counsellors and psychotherapists in the UK practise privately or through charities and voluntary organisations, as availability of counselling and psychotherapy through the NHS is limited and you can wait a long time for a restricted number of sessions.

We know that not all experiences of therapy are positive. We frequently see clients who have previously been disappointed by therapy that proved to be a waste of time and money, and in some cases deeply distressing. In the main, therapy works well, but not *all* therapy works. While 75% of people in the survey mentioned above (BACP, 2019) would recommend therapy to a friend, the remaining 25% presumably would not. That's a lot of people. Similarly, in other research, conducted by the Royal College of Psychiatrists (McQuaid et al., 2021), one in 20 people reported negative effects from their therapy. That's not good enough.

We want to make therapy better. We want to make it work for even more people. We want everyone to know how to avoid wasting money on bad therapy. We want you to be able to get the therapy you need, steer clear of silly fads, cut through jargon and avoid approaches that make no sense. Whether you are currently in therapy, looking for help for a family member or supporting a friend, this book will tell you what your options are, the strengths and weaknesses of different approaches and how to match your problems to a type of therapy and a type of therapist that is right for you.

This book is an insiders' guide to getting the very best help available: a way of ensuring you don't waste money or time on mediocre therapy that falls short of what you need or just isn't for you.

Outline of this book

We begin with a summary of the potential benefits of therapy. Given how expensive therapy with a private, independent practitioner is, we begin by asking the simple question, 'Is it worth it, and how will it help you?' The answer to that depends on what kind of therapy you choose, who you see and what your problem is. So, we encourage you to be questioning throughout this book. While, in the main, therapy helps (Wampold & Imel, 2015), some therapy and some therapists help more than others (Wampold & Brown, 2005). And some therapy won't help at all for some problems (Mayou et al., 2000). So, in the first chapter, we look at the facts and figures, and also at what ordinary people get from therapy, as well as what an ever-growing list of the rich and famous tell the media they got from it.

Chapter 2 considers the practicalities of who's who in the world of mental health more broadly. What's the difference between a psychiatrist, a psychotherapist, a psychologist, a counsellor and a coach? And which is best for you?

Chapter 3 considers what's what – therapy, counselling, psychotherapy, coaching, psychiatry, psychology or psychoanalysis? We describe what you can expect from each approach, and we invite you to take a brief assessment to work out what might suit you and your circumstances best.

In Chapter 4 we focus on how to get the right therapy for you. Teenagers with OCD need a different approach from, say, someone 'feeling stuck' in mid-career or a couple who are constantly arguing. Dealing with addiction requires a different approach from dealing with depression. Some therapists and types of therapy claim to do it all. We consider what treatment delivered by whom is likely to be the most effective for you and your specific issues.

Once you know what type of therapy you want, Chapter 5 helps you choose your therapist and considers what the research says about what constitutes good therapy. We encourage you to ask the therapist questions: about training, their specialist areas of skill and knowledge, their professional qualifications and registration, and how they keep up to date with new research. We suggest you question your therapist as you might a doctor who is about to perform an operation on a loved one: why are they recommending this particular approach and what's their track record in helping people in a similar position? But we also suggest you focus on 'fit': Do they 'get' you? Do you trust them enough to open up to them, and do you believe they are able to help you?

In Chapter 6, we consider how to spot and avoid bad therapy. Most of the hundreds of different types of therapies on offer have not been tested or researched in legitimate trials. Many make ridiculous claims about how they work. And some, as we've already said, can actually make things worse (Mayou et al., 2000). We set out some principles you should apply when making your choice.

Chapters 7 and 8 ask if it's possible to avoid some of the hard emotional work of therapy by using technology and drugs to accelerate change. We consider the use of psychiatric medication, psychedelic-assisted therapy and the escalating emergence of computer-based help and apps. Some say all mental health problems are rooted in a chemical imbalance in the brain and only drugs can help. Others say that medication treats the symptom, not the cause. We provide you with the research and statistics to help you plot your way through this complex terrain, armed with the facts to back up your choices.

Finally, Chapter 9 challenges you to be honest about how serious you are about change. Therapy is hard work. If you're not ready, we suggest that you're probably better off saving your time and money. One of the most important research findings is that what *you* bring to therapy makes the most impact on what you get out of therapy (we'll tell you more about this in Chapter 1). So, we finish with a set of questions that will help you decide if you really are ready to invest the time, money and effort necessary to make therapy work.

We believe that if you do make that investment, you will see the benefit, more often than not. Mental health may be the UK's biggest social problem, but it is chronically under-resourced, and personal therapy is one of the least well-funded areas in our NHS. The sad reality is that often you won't be able to get the help you need from the NHS. In that case, you need to know how to get good quality help elsewhere. That's where this book comes in.

Chapter 1
Why therapy is worth it, and how it will help you

A lot of effort goes into therapy, not least in terms of your time and money. So this chapter sets out what you'll get from therapy and asks whether the effort you need to invest to make therapy work is worth it.

We'll look at recovery rates and satisfaction surveys to help us answer that question. But we'll also consider the people behind the numbers and percentages and see what they get from therapy. In particular, we'll hear what some of the most famous people in the world have to say about their experiences of therapy, from Barack Obama to Harry Styles. And we'll describe the changes in the lives of the ordinary people we see, day in and day out, in our work as therapists.

But before that, we'll summarise what we know about good therapy and tell you what to expect, what to avoid and what you'll need to put into it to make it work.

Good therapy can change your life

We see those changes in our clients. In therapy, you become more accepting of what you may have thought of as your partner's 'flaws' and more realistic about your own. You allow people into your life; you are less selfish, less needy and less demanding. You are less consumed with status, but also more able to accept that it's really quite normal occasionally to be envious of your friends.

You are better able to resolve problems in your life by describing what you want, without drama, exaggeration or threats. You are able to apologise when you're in the wrong and you're more accepting of problems that you just have to live with. Increasingly, you know that feelings come and go and that, while a situation might be unpleasant, it might also only be temporary. You put setbacks into perspective, continue to savour what is good about your life and, when the time is right, you try again.

As well as seeing these changes in our clients, it's what the research shows too. Reviews of research over the past decades (Wampold & Imel, 2015) consistently show that psychotherapy is highly effective – more effective in fact than almost all interventions in cardiology and more effective even than 'flu vaccinations (this can be measured and compared by calculating what in statistics are called 'effect sizes'). In simple terms, three-quarters of people who have therapy end up in a better state of emotional health than those with comparable mental health who don't (Lemma et al., 2011). It's a worthwhile investment of public funds and the reason why the NHS spends £14.3 billion pounds a year on treating mental ill health in England (Baker, 2021). Nearly two million people are referred for NHS therapy each year, and another half a million undertake therapy online (NHS Digital, 2022b).

We also personally know that therapy works because we saw the difference it made in our own lives. It changed us dramatically for the better. But getting good therapy is not as straightforward as you'd suppose.

Getting good therapy can be like crossing a minefield

There are more than 500 types of therapy (Lilienfeld & Arkowitz, 2012) that could be provided by someone calling themselves a psychotherapist, a psychoanalyst, a psychologist, a counsellor or a coach. None of these job titles are defined or protected by law, which means literally anyone can call themselves by any one of them. That's the bad news.

The good news is that most of those practising in any of these roles are likely to be well trained and well intentioned. But you do need to check the relevant statutory registers, or the relevant professional registers overseen by the Professional Standards Authority, to make sure they are who they say they are and are properly qualified to perform what they are offering.

Then there's the decision about which of these professionals is going to be offering the kind of help you need. Each has their area(s) of specialism and particular tools of their trade. No single professional is necessarily any better than another in every circumstance. As we go on to explain in Chapter 2, you might need a psychiatrist to assess you if you are suffering from paranoid or psychotic thoughts and would benefit from medication to calm you down, but detailed knowledge of psychotropic drugs is unlikely to be very useful if you're seeking to rebuild your life after a relationship breakdown has left you devastated or your life partner has suddenly died.

In general, you should choose a treatment that has a sound evidence base and makes sense to you. Do your research first: cognitive behavioural therapy (CBT), psychoanalysis and person-centred counselling are all quite different approaches with different kinds of evidence to prove they can work. Be wary of fads. Therapy is prone to them. As a rule of thumb, if it's not endorsed and offered by the NHS, think very carefully about whether it is right for you. At best, you'll be paying for something that is unproven. At worst, you're paying for something that amounts to snake oil. Hold that in mind for now, as we'll have much more to say about evidence in Chapter 4.

And remember, all *good* therapy has much in common: it looks a lot alike, works in a similar way and is effective to about the same extent (Wampold & Imel, 2015). So if you're choosing a mainstream therapy that makes sense to you and is being delivered by a qualified professional, then the chances are it will help. As we've said, it works for more than 75% of people who get therapy (Lemma et al., 2011).

Your preferences matter

It might seem as if there should be just one optimal type of treatment for each particular problem, but there is currently no single type of therapy that works for everyone with any one mental health condition (Layard & Clark, 2015a). That means that you are going to have to choose.

We also know, from multiple studies, that you are more likely to have a positive outcome if you have chosen a therapy that you believe in and think will work for you (Cooper et al., 2017). So take your preferences seriously and weigh them alongside what the research says works best for your particular problem.

Bear in mind too that the National Institute for Health and Care Excellence (more handily known as NICE), the independent body that evaluates and makes recommendations to the NHS about which are the most effective health and social care treatments, makes no recommendations whatsoever for many of the most common issues we encounter in our day-to-day lives – like relationship problems, anger management or feeling lonely, 'stuck' or inadequate in your job. For these very common and often major life issues, you'll need to choose the type of therapy that makes sense to you and that you are most likely to stick with.

Choose your therapist carefully

If you decide to see a private therapist and pay for therapy, you'll also have to choose the therapist (in the NHS and voluntary sector, you are unlikely to have that luxury; you'll get whoever is employed by the organisation and available). The research tells us that good therapy can't be separated from the therapist who delivers it. Good therapy and good therapists are two sides of the same coin. Different therapists get very different results (Wampold & Brown, 2005; Kraus et al., 2016). So choosing the right therapist may determine whether you get the help you need or not (Owen et al., 2019).

And it's not just about training and qualifications; it's about the person too. Research (Eubanks & Goldfried, 2019) suggests that the best therapists have very particular qualities: they are empathic, non-judgemental, affirming, genuine, focused on your goals, hopeful, solution-focused and willing to act as a guide. Even then, what works for one person won't necessarily work for another. So, once again, bear in mind your preferences. If you know that some qualities are more important to you than others, factor them into your choice. How you get on with your therapist plays a significant role in the outcome of therapy (Ardito & Rabellino, 2011). Do they seem to 'get' you, and do you trust them?

When making your choice, use directory sites that list qualified therapists who are accredited by and registered with a recognised professional or statutory body. You can also use the therapist's own description (on their directory listing or their own website, if they have one) to get a 'feel' for them. Make use of any initial, brief (often free) introductory call that most therapists offer (this is different from an initial assessment, which should come later, once you've contracted for sessions). If the interaction feels positive, go ahead and book your first session. But don't be afraid to move on if you need to. And remember, your therapist doesn't need to be perfect; good enough is good enough.

Good therapy depends on your genuine expectation that it will help. That requires you to have confidence in your therapist. Therapy will improve your awareness of what is going on in your life and how your mind works. You'll see how you typically relate to others and when you tend to overreact or become impulsive or inflexible. Therapy is an opportunity to make deliberate choices to act differently. In very simple terms, it helps you increase your awareness of the things you want to change and notice when you are on autopilot, and it then encourages you to make a decision to do something differently.

While the stereotype of psychotherapy is that it focuses on the past and your childhood and how that has shaped the person you are now, a good therapist will also encourage you to put your emphasis on living your life now, in the present. Looking back to how the past has had an impact on us is often helpful. But good therapy also looks at the things you want to do more of, what's already working and how you build on that.

If good food is a combination of good quality ingredients and the skill of the chef who combines them, then good therapy is a combination of useful techniques and the skill of the therapist who applies them. Decades of research (Miller & Moyers, 2021) suggest that a good therapist is someone you trust and with whom you feel comfortable and have a connection. Therapy is hard. Don't make it harder by choosing someone you don't get on with and don't respect.

Avoid bad therapy like the plague

If you aren't happy with your therapist or what they are offering, don't just put up with it. Even if you have chosen a therapist who is registered with one of the main regulatory bodies and a member of a recognised professional association, use your common sense too: if your therapist is often late for appointments or leaves you feeling awful after every session, look elsewhere. If they lack humility or dismiss your feedback when you raise complaints or concerns, choose someone else. If they are not helping you feel better, raise that with them and talk about the reasons why together. If they won't do that, or make you feel uncomfortable when you do so, then that of itself is a reason to go elsewhere.

Remain open to the likelihood that therapy will help you, but retain a healthy scepticism about inflated promises, especially in relation to new types of therapy. Focus on types of therapy for which there is good evidence and that have stood the test of time.

There is no silver bullet

Therapy hasn't changed much in more than a century, but some recent innovations are worth noting. Current research suggests that online therapy works as well as in-person therapy (Batastini et al., 2020). The Covid-19 pandemic gave a huge boost to online individual therapy, which had been regarded with suspicion before it became the only kind possible during lockdowns. But people nowadays expect a different kind of engagement with healthcare, especially if they are paying for it. There's been considerable investment by some big international organisations in providing types of online therapy that are cheaper, more accessible and more in the client's control than traditional weekly face-to-face sessions. Some allow you to message a therapist out of hours and give you the ability to change therapists whenever you want to.

Both sound good in theory. Being able to change therapists is great when things are genuinely not working. But therapy is also about encouraging you to step outside your comfort zone and confront avoidance and excuses. If your therapist is gently challenging you, it is likely to feel uncomfortable but it's most definitely not a reason to find another one who is more accommodating to your wishes. Similarly, having your therapist on call at any time of night or day might actually cut across your ability to learn to tolerate anxiety and make your own decisions.

NICE guidance tells us that antidepressants can be beneficial for a lot of people with moderate and severe depression and generalised anxiety, but should not be used for milder kinds of depression, where therapy is your best option (NICE, 2022). There is growing interest in psychedelic-assisted therapy, but at time of writing, the research isn't strong enough to recommend it yet.

Often people look to drugs and technology to short-cut the process of therapy or to save money. But if money really is the issue, you're better off seeking low-fee therapy (for example, via local charity providers) or using the computer-based cognitive behavioural options provided by the NHS, which are available via self-referral. Or you could buy yourself an evidence-based self-help therapy workbook and apply the ideas – we recommend some in 'Further Reading and Resources' at the end of the book. Therapy is expensive but the cost is relative. What else might you spend that money on that is worth more than your mental wellbeing? You wouldn't choose your solicitor or accountant solely on the basis of who was least expensive. As in most areas of life, you usually get what you pay for.

To make therapy work, you'll have to work – hard!

Good therapy and a good therapist are critical to getting a good outcome from therapy. But your motivation and readiness matter more. Research tells us that it's the factors you bring to therapy, such as your history, interpersonal skills and motivation, that determine how likely therapy is to work (Lambert, 2013).

This ought not to be a great surprise. In every field of human endeavour, effort counts. You get out what you put in. Therapy is no different. If you turn up late, aren't honest about what you're feeling and constantly blame others, you won't get much out of it.

That doesn't mean you have to be the 'perfect client', 100% ready to change, though. There are many stages on the journey to change. You need to recognise the things you want to change, which ones will be easier and which harder and the order to take them in, and weigh up the emotional as well as financial cost and whether it's worth it. If it is, you need to work out the best way of making those changes. Then, of course, you need to take those actions and monitor how well this is working. And along the way, you need to keep going when it's difficult, bounce back when you slip up or fall back, lock those changes into a new way of life and maintain them. Easy to say, not to do.

Changing behaviour is difficult and time consuming. Neuroscience tells us that the brain can change but, like the muscles in your body, it takes time and consistent effort. The key is to take action even when you don't feel like it. A good therapist can help at every stage of the process, but they can't do the work for you.

So, bearing all that in mind, is therapy worth it?

The numbers and the statistics suggest therapy is worth it. There are several tried and tested treatments for which there is considerable and well-respected research showing they work. Those treatments are subject to the same rigorous tests (Layard & Clark, 2015a) as those used to test treatments for physical illness, and – as we've said – the success rates are just as high (Lemma et al., 2011). Changes brought about by therapy can be seen via brain imaging (Linden, 2006). Improvements also show up in the number of hours slept, or the number of days spent panic free. In one study (Eisler et al., 2000), clients with anorexia weighed on average eight kilograms more after 12 months of therapy. In these instances, therapy can be the literal difference between life and death.

But let's go beyond the numbers and look at the people behind the percentages. Everyone is having therapy these days. From Bruce Springsteen to Barack and Michelle Obama; from Adele to Pope Francis. Many of those famous people have had profound experiences of therapy and talk openly, in life-changing terms, about their experiences. We consider a few below.

The music legend Bruce Springsteen has had decades of struggle with depression and even suicidal thoughts at one point. He first started seeing a therapist in the early 1980s and has continued to do so throughout his long career (Greene, 2012).

The former US First Lady, Michelle Obama opened up about going to couples counselling, saying that she was 'one of those wives who thought they were taking their husband to marriage counselling so he could be fixed'. Instead, she says, the spotlight fell on her too, forcing her to realise she wasn't perfect. Marriage counselling was a 'turning point', she says (Nechamkin, 2018).

Tennis champion Serena Williams reached out for help from a therapist after her half-sister was murdered in 2003 (Williams & Paisner, 2009). She got help again following the 2018 US Open final. She says seeing a therapist helped her work through her feelings about how women in public life are expected to deal with their emotions (Aggeler, 2019).

Even Pope Francis has had therapy. Six months of therapy during his younger years helped him to understand his anxiety and manage his fears, and he continues to use the techniques he learned then (Sherwood & Giuffrida, 2017).

Rapper Jay-Z told the *New York Times* that therapy played a crucial part in repairing his marriage to Beyoncé (Baquet, 2017). Singer Adele says that therapy helped her deal with both her father's death and, later, her divorce (Aguirre, 2021). Singer Harry Styles said of his decision to start weekly therapy: 'I felt like I exercise every day and take care of my body, so why wouldn't I do that with my mind?' (Spanos, 2022). Actors Emma Thompson (Nikkhah, 2010), Keira Knightley (Millea, 2015) and Sophie Turner (Hiatt & Nodland, 2019) all commend it.

The list of celebrities who describe how therapy helped goes on and on: Stephen Fry, Halle Berry, Brad Pitt, Brooke Shields, Michael B. Jordan, Simone Biles, Demi Lovato, Robert Downey Jr, Catherine Zeta-Jones, Ruby Wax, Richard Osman, Alex Scott, Hugh Laurie, Jon Hamm, Michael Phelps, Danny Rose and Anne-Marie. Justin Bieber even posted a picture of himself in a therapy session, captioned, 'Therapy session, it's cool to have a healthy mind and healthy emotions' (cited in Goldstein, 2019).

But what about 'real' people – what do they say about therapy? Are they just as positive? Well, at the headline level, we know that 75% of them are better off and would recommend therapy (BACP, 2019). But what about the specific changes as a consequence of therapy? What do they do differently as a result? And what benefits might you therefore expect? In other words, is therapy worth it?

What follow are some of the most important benefits that clients we see get from therapy, week in, week out. We feel confident to predict that theirs is not a unique experience.

Spot your patterns and automatic defaults

You learn to see what you previously couldn't. You start to see the wood for the trees. You recognise your patterns, automatic defaults, tendencies, core beliefs or narratives. Whatever you call them, the stories that you have constructed about yourselves are the lens through which you see the world and interpret events.

Therapy helps you recognise your automatic thoughts, the assumptions that underlie them and your core beliefs.

Perhaps you feel like you can't rely on your partner and you are constantly afraid they may leave you. You assume that relationships are unstable and likely to lead to abandonment. Or maybe you feel some shame, that you are defective in some way, which results in you thinking that, if your partner saw 'the real you', they would leave. Or perhaps your pattern has more to do with entitlement. As a consequence, you get angry when you don't get what you want from your partner, and you complain about this or try to manipulate them into doing things your way.

However those tendencies play out, the familiar patterns are what you *do*, but they are not who you *are*. They are defaults, but they can be reset. Once you see them for what they are, it's up to you whether you keep acting on them or not.

Realise that it's not your fault

Part of the purpose of therapy is to help you understand why you have those tendencies. Therapy helps you understand how and why you are the way you are: a mix of your genetic inheritance and your life experiences to date.

If you didn't get a healthy dose of care and attention while growing up, you may well have an underdeveloped sense of self-esteem. If you weren't accepted and respected, and if you weren't allowed to express yourself, you may well have difficulty expressing your wants and needs now. You might assume your feelings don't matter or will be dismissed by others, and therefore you might not bother asking for things you want or need. Alternatively, you might be extremely demanding, assuming others will only respond if you compel or manipulate them.

Similarly, if you haven't been set realistic limits in childhood, or haven't been taught self-control and respect for others, then you will likely end up treating others poorly. If you have been over-indulged as a child, you can easily grow up not understanding the need to consider other people before acting. In the absence of realistic limits and concern for others, you may well have a strong sense of your own entitlement or grandiosity.

To realise that these tendencies come from somewhere is helpful. It stops you blaming yourself. That doesn't mean you automatically blame your parents instead! They may have been at fault. But they may have also been doing their best. Of course, in some cases of abuse and neglect, you may rightly need to hold your parents, or other adults, responsible for what they did or didn't do. But in others, perhaps less severe, therapy helps you realise that it's okay to say you were treated in a way you didn't want to be, or that you missed out on important things you needed in childhood, but that you don't need to blame anyone else for that.

Take responsibility and ask for what you want

This is a key point about therapy, which is often missed. It's about taking responsibility for yourself. It may not be your fault, but it is your responsibility to take action and break the cycle if you want a better life. Insight into why you are the way you are is the first step, but it doesn't get you very far on its own. If you want things to be different, you will have to do more than notice your patterns and defaults: you'll have to *do* something about them. You will have to change your behaviour.

If you want your life to change, you will have to start to ask for what you want, share your feelings openly and learn how to listen, negotiate and compromise with others. It's no good saying you had a tough start in life and therefore this is the way you are. You can and should assert your point of view, but your attitude to the other person also needs to be respectful if you want a decent relationship with them. If you want to live well around other people, you will have to acknowledge and respect their wants and feelings, as well as your own.

Stop seeing the world in black and white or catastrophic terms

Linked to the need to do things differently is the need to think differently. It is easier said than done, but not impossible. Therapy will help you challenge longstanding tendencies to see situations as all or nothing. Your boss is an idiot, you do all the childcare, your partner never listens, your kids are inconsiderate, your parents always have to have the last word. Therapy questions statements that contain 'never' or 'always', because they are seldom true. Therapy invites you to notice and change your tone and moderate your thinking and language where it is accusatory, argumentative, self-pitying or categorical.

In therapy, you begin to see shades of grey. You stop seeing the world in all-or-nothing terms. You stop over-generalising or jumping to conclusions that aren't warranted by the facts. You stop assuming you know what other people are thinking. You stop demanding that things 'should' or 'must' be a certain way. You stop making negative predictions about the future, and instead you wait and see. You stop blowing things out of proportion, magnifying conflicts or catastrophising situations. Many situations will continue to be frustrating and annoying, but therapy helps you see that, more often than not, you can cope, and even thrive, in spite of them.

See emotions as useful

Emotions are not an inconvenience or a nuisance. You don't need to be afraid of them, even the 'negative' ones. They are there to tell you something. They are useful. Your feelings are not to be dismissed, wished away or ignored. They have meaning and can prompt you to take action when you otherwise might not. Sadness shows you how much you want a situation to be better. Loneliness prompts you to connect more with the people in your life, rekindle old relationships or forge new ones. Feelings of frustration tell you that you want more from life. Anxiety keeps you vigilant and ensures you take care of what you've got and that you continue to work hard on what's important to you. The physiological arousal and urgency associated with anger gives you the energy and courage to protect the things you care about.

Feelings are a fact of life. They are a reminder that you are made of flesh and blood. They cannot be wished away or turned off. Therapy helps you consider the functions of emotions: without anger, you might not act; without frustration, you might not drive yourself on; without fear, you might not take steps to avoid danger. Athletes and performers don't try to get rid of anxiety and nerves: they use them as a source of energy and focus. Therapy teaches you to check in with your feelings and see when they are telling you something important.

Accept the things that can't be changed

Of course, there are times when emotions run away with you. The brain is evolved to keep you alive; its job is to scan for danger and risk, not to keep you happy (Euba, 2019). That can result in you feeling afraid, fearful and anxious a lot of the time, if you're not careful. Not all the danger signals the brain sends you are useful and not every situation you face is life threatening. You can use your mind to filter those signals, take action when needed, and moderate your responses when they are over the top, or simply live with them.

Working out exactly the right choice in different circumstances requires judgement. As the old saying goes, sometimes we need the serenity to accept the things that can't be changed; sometimes we need the courage to change the things that can, and we always need the wisdom to know the difference. There are times when emotions don't serve you well (public speaking is not improved by you having a dry mouth or being breathless through sheer terror). In those cases, you can remind yourself that you are not in mortal danger; that the most likely outcome is not that you will make a fool of yourself or be ostracised from the group, and that most people in the audience wish you well and will have experienced those exact same feelings themselves.

Some of the most useful advice is just to accept difficult feelings and do what matters most in that situation, regardless. That might mean asking someone out when you are nervous, contributing an important point to a discussion at work, or giving a speech at a friend's wedding even when it makes you anxious to do so.

More generally, you don't always have to take everything in life so seriously. The things you often attach to – money, prestige, the opinion of others, being seen as a good person – don't matter as much as you think. Nor do the stories you tell yourself about who you should be or what your life should be like. The consequence of adopting a more accepting stance in relation to your endless stream of preferences and preoccupations is that they will trouble you less. While there are things worth changing about yourself, you are a human being, we are all variously flawed, and you are not likely to transcend human nature. This is the way to psychological health.

In therapy, you learn not to spin out about unwanted thoughts and feelings. You begin to see them as inevitable. Life is full of difficult bosses, annoying neighbours, stress, worry, anxiety, irritation, partners who disappoint you and children who aren't sufficiently grateful. How you respond is what matters. You are nervous before you give a talk in public, but you can still give the talk. You don't like large gatherings, but the occasion is important to your partner, so you go. Your children don't always appreciate what you do for them, but you continue to love them and look after them anyway.

In all of those situations, you can notice what's going on inside your head and make a decision about how to respond, based on your longer-term values. Let's say your partner is late home from a work function. You are generally quick to catastrophise: being late means they don't care about you – or maybe they've had an accident. But if you can slow down that thought process, you can see that you don't have to send an accusatory text, involve other family members in your panic or sulk when they finally get in. You can send them a text letting them know you are worried about them. If you don't get a response and you think they've been unreasonable, you can talk about it the following day. And sometimes you can just let it go. They lost track of time and were back later than expected, but they are safely home now. Sometimes stuff is not such a big deal.

Build resilience

Often the everyday problems of life are best resolved via our natural resilience and the healing powers of time. We don't always have to act. We are a tough species, the successful survivors of 10,000 generations of resourceful ancestors who lived with hunger and who dealt with dangers beyond our imagination (Frances, 2013).

Therapy will help you to see that you are stronger than you think. Therapy will challenge your tendency to find fault, fuss, worry that you can't cope or fear the worst. In therapy, you learn to stop clinging, withdrawing, attacking, seeking reassurance, giving reassurance, defending, controlling or demanding. Instead, you develop more confidence in yourself and your judgements and you learn communication skills based on asserting your wants and preferences. In short, therapy builds new ways of behaving based on your in-built resilience.

Learning to express yourself honestly in a way that is clear and unapologetic allows others to hear what you want without being overwhelmed. Stating your preferences clearly and briefly, without accusations, means you are more likely to be heard and understood. Therapy helps you stand up for your rights without anger, without acting in an intimidating, controlling, manipulating or needy manner.

Doing that takes courage and is likely to feel alien at first. Learning any new skill is difficult. Therapy helps you notice, nurture and reinforce the progress you are making as you try out new things. In time, many of those new ways of thinking, speaking and acting will become second nature. Until then, therapy is often the right place to practise them.

Risking exposure and facing the unknown

Changing your behaviour means stepping into the unknown, and that is bound to be uncomfortable. Asking your partner for something that is important to you but that they might not want to give you or asking someone out on a date will make you feel anxious and vulnerable. Asking for more money at work, confronting a difficult co-worker or telling your partner that you are leaving a dysfunctional relationship will result in uncomfortable feelings in the short term. Therapy helps you see that facing difficult situations and the feelings they bring up is the price of admission to a good life.

Deliberately and repeatedly doing what you're afraid of reduces that fear in time too, and sometimes even eventually extinguishes it. Confronting a difficult situation or person allows you to realise that it wasn't so bad or, at the very least, you survived it. Sometimes you even get what you want. Avoiding things that cause you anxiety, such as going to parties, getting on a plane or driving on a busy motorway, may produce less anxiety in the short term, but in the long run it means your anxiety is maintained. Every time you avoid something, you reinforce the sense that it is a big deal and it really is scary. At the same time, you diminish your life by limiting the things you feel you can do.

The presence of difficult thoughts or feelings is not the problem; the problem comes when you treat those thoughts and feelings very seriously: as truths or rules that must be followed or obeyed. But if you can detach from those thoughts and realise that they do not need to be taken so seriously or immediately acted on, you become free to choose a course of action guided by your values and longer-term aims.

Psychological flexibility

You might notice that sometimes we are saying 'Stand up for yourself', and at other times we are inviting you to 'let things go' because they might not matter so much. Similarly, sometimes we are saying, 'Tune into your feelings' and use them to take action, and at other times we are saying, 'You don't always have to take your feelings (or yourself) so seriously'. That's because, above all else, therapy aims to give you the freedom and flexibility to choose.

Being psychologically flexible is the key to a good life. Adaptation is the defining trait of the human race, and therapy helps you think and act flexibly. It helps you take a realistic view of the situation, balance your short- and long-term interests and weigh up your needs alongside the needs of others. Life is complex, sometimes contradictory and always changing. Obstacles appear and plans change; people let you down; friends move away; you get passed over for promotion; your partner leaves you; you fall in love; a loved one dies; you get a job offer in another country; your child starts refusing to go to school; you inherit money; you suffer an accident or illness; your boss moves on and you are asked to take over; you fail important exams; you are made redundant. The list goes on.

Being flexible allows you to respond to ever-changing circumstances. Being rigid or inflexible leads to all sorts of problems. When you're experiencing strong emotions, it's easy to assume that these feelings alone should guide your behaviour. Psychological flexibility allows you to have those strong feelings and still be able to apply rational thought to the situation, all the while drawing on your longer-term values. Putting all that together means that you can do what matters most. That *might* still mean giving someone a piece of your mind, but it more likely will allow you to see that there might be something more important at stake. Psychological flexibility means your behaviour is not based on just your peak emotions at one moment in time.

Psychological inflexibility and the inability to see things in the round is at the root of many of the actions you later regret: angry emails, harsh words to friends, office affairs, rash spending choices, walking away in fear from a situation where you needed to stand firm. Too often, in the presence of strong feelings, we become narrow and rigid in our responses. Psychological flexibility means being able to respond to what is actually in front of you, not what you would like to be in front of you. It means noticing your old automatic ways and focusing on doing the next right thing, guided by your longer-term values.

Therapy helps you with all aspects of life

You may enter therapy to resolve relationship conflict with your partner and then find that the insight, tools and techniques for doing so can be applied to a host of other situations. Such techniques might make you a more thoughtful manager or a better negotiator; they might mean you can step back from the shouting matches you sometimes get into with your children.

Or let's say you come to therapy to explore how your childhood and your parents' stormy marriage continue to influence the way you behave in your marriage today. In the process of doing that, you are likely to learn about how you deal with criticism, which could apply equally in a work setting, where giving and receiving feedback is a regular occurrence and where opportunities for judgement and evaluation (of yourself and others) are frequent.

Some of the simple but fundamental ideas you encounter in therapy translate into many areas of life. Dealing with catastrophic thoughts about a relationship ('My partner is going to leave me') can equally be applied to negative thought spirals about finances or whether you will ever become pregnant. How you notice and then challenge all-or-nothing thinking is the same, whether they are thoughts about how supposedly worthless you are, thoughts about what an utter idiot your boss is or worries about money.

Summing it up

Given the above, our view is that therapy is both well worth it and far too important to simply hope for the best or take pot luck. It enables you to see when you're on autopilot, mindlessly repeating old patterns. It helps you take responsibility for yourself and no longer blame others for your problems. It encourages you to take more calculated risks, leave behind the feeling that you're not good enough, question your attachments to money and status, and reconnect with the things that matter most. And it means doing so with courage, resilience and an ability to weather the tough times, as you pursue what is most important to you in life.

We are pro-therapy, on the basis of our experience as therapists and clients and on the basis of the research evidence. But we encourage you to be discerning and sometimes even sceptical when making choices about what sort of therapy you look for and what sort of therapist you choose. There are often life-changing benefits from getting good therapy, but there is also bad therapy and average therapy, just as there are therapists who will really help you and therapists you should probably avoid.

It would be far simpler if therapy were freely available on the NHS. But that's not even remotely the case. Nor is it likely to be any time soon: one-to-one therapy is far too expensive. That's why GPs are compelled to prescribe antidepressants in the numbers they do: they have very few other treatments to offer. That's why more and more people are seeking therapy outside the NHS. But to do so, you need to know what to look for, so you don't waste your time and money and you don't miss out on the life-changing benefits of good therapy.

The rest of the book tells you how to get good therapy. Before you read on, below are the 10 most important things we think you need to remember from this chapter. Bear them in mind as you continue reading about how to get yourself the kind of therapy that can change your life for the better.

Ten things to remember

1. Three-quarters of people who've had therapy say it was worth it. And an estimated three-quarters of people who have therapy are better off subsequently than those who don't.
2. Most ordinary people don't speak publicly about the benefits of therapy. But when celebrities do, almost all of them – from Pope Francis to Harry Styles – say it changed their life. You can reasonably expect this too.
3. Therapy helps you spot your automatic patterns, understand where they come from, take responsibility for them and change the way you think and act.

4. Therapy helps you see emotions as useful and notice their function: without anger you might not have the courage to act; without frustration, you might not drive yourself on.
5. Athletes and performers harness their emotions to improve their performance. Therapy helps you to do the same.
6. Therapy encourages you to accept the things you can't change. Unwanted thoughts, feelings and situations are inevitable. Life is full of difficulties.
7. Everyday problems are often best resolved by using your natural resilience. We are a tough species. Therapy helps you realise that you're stronger and more resilient than you think.
8. Psychological flexibility is the key to a good life. Being flexible means responding to what is in front of you, not what you'd like to be in front of you or what you fear is in front of you. Therapy helps you think and act flexibly.
9. The benefits of therapy can be applied across many areas of life. The insights and techniques you learn to work through issues with your partner can serve you equally well with your boss, your co-workers, your clients or your kids.
10. For most people, most of the time and with most problems, therapy works and is worth the time, effort and expense involved.

Chapter 2
Who's who?

Not only are there more than 500 different types of therapy; they could also be delivered by someone calling themselves a psychotherapist, a psychoanalyst, a psychologist, a counsellor or a coach. And to make matters even more complex, none of those roles are legally defined or protected. That means anyone can call themselves by any one of those titles without having had a single day of training.

So how to know where to start? How do you know which of these therapists and which therapy might be best for you? And how do you avoid being ripped off? Let's start by explaining who's who, and how to make sure you're getting help from someone who is properly trained and qualified.

In this book we use the term 'therapist' to include anyone who is practising therapy (that could be any of the professionals listed in this section). But there are some big differences between them: not only what they do, how they practise and the kinds of therapy/treatments they offer, but also what they charge, where and what they have studied and for how long, and where they are based. They might work from a wood-panelled office in a smart part of town, for example, or in an NHS hospital department, or in the spare room of their own home.

You might assume that, if you can afford it, the one that costs the most and has the smartest office and their own receptionist is therefore better than the others. But who is likely to help you most really depends on your needs. If you need a formal diagnosis and medication, then you most likely need a psychiatrist. But they are unlikely to be your best option if you are coming to terms with a bereavement, if you and your partner need help resolving conflicts in your relationship or if you feel stuck in your career.

So, as you read the descriptions below, bear in mind the differences and similarities between the roles and keep in mind your particular problem as you think about who is best placed to help you.

Psychotherapist/therapist

Most likely, if you see a psychotherapist, you'll see them privately, meaning you're paying out of your own pocket and having your sessions at a private clinic, training institute or in their home. If referred via your GP, you may see a psychotherapist at a GP surgery, local health centre or an outpatient clinic at a hospital. Most private therapists offer open-ended therapy, meaning they'll work with you for as long as it takes to reach your goals; there'll be no limit on the number of sessions, other than how many you can afford. Most NHS therapy treatment, by contrast, is limited in terms of the number of sessions you'll have with your therapist – typically between eight and 20 (NHS, 2022b).

Your therapist is likely to dress in smart-casual clothes and work from an environment that is designed to be warm, comfortable and put you at ease. The first few sessions are likely to involve an exploration of why you're seeking help at this time in your life, what you're struggling with and why you're in distress. Sessions are usually 50 minutes to an hour and start and end promptly.

Over time, your therapist will likely agree some goals for the therapy with you. Some therapists emphasise this more than others, and some try to establish that as the focus for therapy early on. Others allow it to emerge more slowly. Many therapists will work with you to develop a plan based on how they will try to help you, and some will write that down and give it to you. Others will see that as happening more naturally, and will take their lead from you. Your therapist will likely assess and revise any plan with you during your work together. The plan is likely to involve a mix of talking about your difficulties and how your life experiences contributed to them; your goals and values; tolerating difficult feelings and thoughts sometimes, plus some good ideas to take the edge off intense feelings or some suggestions for trying out new ways of thinking, behaving and feeling.

Some therapists will give you activities to do outside the session: worksheets to complete, for example, or tasks to perform, such as talking to a stranger if you suffer with social anxiety, or having a difficult conversation with your partner. Some will help you practise and prepare for this, if you'd find that useful. Some therapists focus less on this and more on what is going on between you and them, as they believe this is the most immediate and helpful way of shedding light on an area of your life or how you behave.

The titles 'psychotherapist' and 'therapist' (and, indeed, counsellor) are often used interchangeably. As mentioned above, these titles are not legally protected terms, so anyone can call themselves a therapist and practise as such. You can reassure yourself that they are trained and qualified by choosing a therapist registered with a regulatory body (such as the Health and Care Professions Council (HCPC)) or with one of the main professional bodies, such as the British Association for Counselling and Psychotherapy (BACP), the UK Council for Psychotherapy (UKCP) or the National Counselling & Psychotherapy Society (NCS), whose registers are accredited by the Professional Standards Authority (PSA). If a psychotherapist or therapist is overseen by a regulatory body or is listed on a register accredited by the PSA, it means that they have undertaken an accredited training, they will be receiving supervision, they will operate in line with an ethical framework and they will be bound by an independent complaints procedure.

Different membership bodies specify different levels of training. So, some therapists will have undertaken extensive training, often for five to six years, following an undergraduate degree, and they are often educated to master's level. But there are also shorter training options, also accredited by professional bodies, that may not require graduate entry. That may not matter to you; if, say, you are coming to terms with a bereavement, emotional warmth, a listening ear and life experience may be more important to you than the therapist's level of qualification. But if you want specialist help with a more complex issue, such as dealing with an eating disorder or obsessive-compulsive thoughts, bear in mind that not every therapist will have been trained to provide that.

Your best bet is to ask a prospective therapist how often they see people with the kind of problem you are facing, whether they are specifically trained to deal with it, and what their success rate looks like. Therapists should be clear with you when they think they can help and, if they think they are not best placed or qualified to do so, they should refer you on. You should be able to expect this from any therapist who is on the register of any of the professional bodies accredited by the PSA, such as UKCP or BACP, or who is registered with a regulatory body, such as the HCPC.

Psychotherapists often come into the profession as a second career, meaning that, on average, they tend to be in the older age brackets. In a recent survey of the membership of BACP, the largest professional body of therapists, 75% were more than 45 years old, more than a third were aged 55 years-plus, and 15% were 65 or older (Xavier, 2020).

Psychotherapists sometimes work in the NHS but most work in private practice. When working privately, they should have professional indemnity insurance, policies on how they manage your information and data that are compliant with UK law, information setting out what you can expect from them and where to complain if things go wrong, plus regular supervision from an experienced member of the profession to help them develop their skills and ensure they are working safely and ethically.

Counsellor

Seeing a counsellor is quite similar to seeing a psychotherapist. They will invite you to talk about your feelings and problems in a safe, confidential setting – usually a room in their house or a counselling centre or charity organisation premises. The basis of counselling is non-directive, non-judgemental listening and empathic understanding. Your counsellor will listen to you and help you find ways to cope with emotional issues in your life. They will help you understand your feelings and thoughts and find your own solutions to problems. Counsellors tend to be non-directive – that is, they won't tell you what to do about your problems; instead, they work from a stance that you are the best person to understand your problem and decide what is best for you. They believe that you are the expert, the answers are already within you, and that compassionate curiosity will help you uncover them.

Confusingly, the term 'counsellor' is often used interchangeably with 'therapist' or 'psychotherapist', and some professionals refer to themselves by all three titles on different occasions. There is no consensus on whether the titles do or should describe distinctly different ways of working and in what ways they differ.

Those who describe themselves solely as counsellors may be indicating that they favour a listening, supportive approach, and may be less likely to guide or challenge you or encourage you to set goals for therapy. The best way to know exactly what their chosen title says about the way the practitioner works is to ask them.

It is likely that someone who calls themselves a counsellor will have completed a shorter, less intensive initial training than someone who has trained as a psychotherapist, and they are more likely to emphasise active listening and helping you to understand how you feel and what you want to do than to offer guidance, advice and challenge. If you are struggling with a specific emotional problem, such as obsessive-compulsive disorder or severe social anxiety, you may prefer to get support from a psychotherapist or psychologist who specialises in treating your condition, rather than see a counsellor.

As with 'psychotherapist', the title of counsellor is not legally protected, so again, check that they are a registered member of one of the professional bodies accredited by the Professional Standards Authority, such as BACP or the NCS.

Psychologist

Going to see a clinical or counselling psychologist is very much like seeing a psychotherapist. You'll be invited to talk about your difficulties, or 'symptoms', and they will likely agree with you on a plan, or 'treatment plan', which they may suggest to you. It is more likely that a psychologist will follow a medical model and talk in terms of symptoms, treatment plans and interventions. They are likely to focus on developing a plan that uses recognised evidence-based interventions (i.e. those supported by current research findings). You may see an NHS psychologist in an outpatient setting, but many work privately, so you might consult them in a private clinic or at their home. Many clinical psychologists have a specialism, such as obsessive-compulsive disorder or eating disorders, so this might be a good option for you if you have a specific issue in your life or set of symptoms for which you need help and support.

A psychologist will have completed a doctorate in either counselling psychology or clinical psychology. There is considerable overlap between the two roles. Traditionally, counselling psychologists focused on less distressed people and clinical psychologists on people with more serious mental health issues. However, in practice, often both work with similar clients in similar settings.

Psychologists do not have medical training so cannot prescribe medication. While the titles 'clinical psychologist' and 'counselling psychologist' are legally protected, the title 'psychologist' on its own is not, meaning anyone can use it if they choose. Qualified clinical or counselling psychologists will be registered with the Health and Care Professions Council (HCPC) and you can check their registration online.

Psychoanalyst

Psychoanalysts tend to see people several times a week over a long period of time – often many years.

If you see an analyst, you may lie on a couch with the analyst sitting behind you, rather than facing you – the traditional stereotype. This is intended to free the client (often called 'patient' in psychoanalysis) to explore their inner unconscious thoughts with the minimum of distractions from their immediate surroundings. Some say Freud introduced it because he didn't like being stared at all day by his clients. However, some analysts nowadays use facing chairs, like a counsellor or psychotherapist. You'll be invited to explore your unconscious by talking about what's on your mind and following wherever this takes you, with the analyst's support. Because of analysts' interest in the unconscious, you are more likely than you are in other types of therapy to be encouraged to talk about your dreams and fantasies. Analysis is also much less likely to be less goal-orientated than other types of therapy. It gives you the freedom to explore your own mind. You'll do the vast majority of the talking and there may be sessions where your analyst says almost nothing.

Partly due to its cost, the long-term commitment required and the relatively few empirical studies into its effectiveness, psychoanalysis is a relatively rare form of treatment these days and is not available on the NHS, except in much briefer forms. There are around 500 members of the British Psychoanalytic Society, in contrast to the more than 60,000 members of BACP, the largest professional body for counsellors and therapists in the UK.

There is no set time limit for how long it takes to qualify as a psychoanalyst but typically they train for four to five years, following an undergraduate degree. Many will also have a master's degree, although this is not a requirement. The title 'psychoanalyst' is not legally protected either. The members' register of the British Psychoanalytic Council is accredited by the PSA, which guarantees that members have completed an accredited course, including having undergone their own psychoanalysis.

Psychiatrist

Only a minority of people reading this book will need to see a psychiatrist. If you see one, you're likely seeking a formal diagnosis and medication for a severe mental health condition. Although you might well talk with a psychiatrist about the origins of your symptoms and coping strategies, the psychiatrist will focus on treating your symptoms through medication. They may take a physical examination and check your blood pressure to rule out any physical origins of your mental distress. If a psychiatrist feels you need additional psychological or emotional support, they may refer you to a psychotherapist, clinical psychologist or counsellor.

Psychiatrists are qualified medical doctors, so it typically takes 10 years to complete their training. Because of their medical training, psychiatrists are able to do things other mental health professionals can't, such as prescribe medication and carry out blood tests or scans. To call yourself a psychiatrist, you have to have completed the medical training and be registered with the General Medical Council (GMC). You can check if someone is a registered psychiatrist on the GMC website.[1]

Your GP can refer you to see a psychiatrist if they think you may have a severe mental health problem and require medical help. Most psychiatrists work in hospitals or with community mental health teams. If you are referred by your GP, you are likely to be assessed by another less senior member of the mental health team first. Their job is to decide if you need to see a psychiatrist.

---

1. www.gmc-uk.org/registration-and-licensing

There are fewer than 8000 consultant psychiatrists in the UK (Royal College of Psychiatrists, 2021a), meaning you are likely to face a long waiting list before you get to see one, even if you are assessed as needing to do so.

Many psychiatrists also work in private practice, so you can ask your GP to write a referral letter and then pay to see a psychiatrist privately. This is an expensive option but significantly reduces the waiting time. The average initial consultation (usually about 90 minutes) in London can cost in excess of £1000.

But bear in mind that psychiatrists specialise in medicine and may actually have less experience in delivering therapy than many of the other professionals described here. Unless you specifically need medication or a formal psychiatric diagnosis, you may be paying for expertise you don't need.

One area where psychiatrists are particularly in demand is from parents looking for help with their children, who they worry are displaying symptoms associated with ADHD or autism. A formal diagnosis by a psychiatrist is often a necessary passport to treatment and educational and welfare support. As with adults, the referral route is via your GP and a long wait to see an NHS psychiatrist, or dodge the waiting list and pay to see a psychiatrist privately.

Coaches

Coaching is an increasingly popular form of psychological help. Generally associated with sports and other kinds of performance, and with the workplace, 'life coaching' has burgeoned in recent years as more and more people seek advice on how to live healthier, happier and more productive lives. Although there are differences between therapy and coaching, there is also a lot of cross-over, especially between some forms of short-term, problem-solving therapy and 'developmental' or psychological coaching. If you're struggling to make up your mind about a potential career change, how best to manage your workplace team or how to transition into and fulfill a more senior role, seeing a coach might be your best bet. A lot of people see coaches for such work-related matters (usually called 'executive coaches'), but many people benefit from conversations with coaches about wider life challenges, such as chronic procrastination, poor time management or finding a new direction in their life. These are usually called 'life coaches'. Coaches often work with whole organisations or teams, as well as with individuals.

Generally, coaches help people who are experiencing problems that are not related to mental illness or emotional distress. Coaches generally have not been trained to recognise or work with mental ill health or distress and will not want to step outside the boundaries of their professional expertise. Sometimes clients do not know whether their problems are rooted in mental health issues. For this reason, some people like to see practitioners who are qualified therapists *and* coaches, which allows flexibility within sessions. It is quite common now for coaches to have added therapy training to their coaching foundation (and therapists to train as coaches). This means they can switch focus within and between sessions, or take some time working out where their focus should be and engage with problems that relate to work or career progression but also have a psychological component.

Despite a protracted campaign by the main coaching associations, such as the International Coaching Federation (ICF) and the European Mentoring and Coaching Council (EMCC), coaching is almost entirely unregulated. For example, there is no independent government-appointed body (equivalent to the Professional Standards Authority) with powers to oversee the registers of the coaching bodies, as exists for psychotherapy or counselling. Given this, you should take particular care to check your coach's credentials: ask about their training, their expertise and experience, which professional body they belong to, and how they're supervised in their work.

Other titles

The professions listed above are the main titles in use. Sometimes a therapist may add the title of their mode or model of practice, such as cognitive behavioural therapist or person-centred counsellor. This simply means they use that form of therapy. But if someone is using a very specific title that you do not understand, and which is not listed here in this book (such as 'somatic/body-based therapist' or Gestalt, relational or schema therapist, for example), ask them to explain it to you. If they can't explain it in simple terms, move on. You need to work with someone who can explain in plain English what they do and how they work. If they are unclear, evasive, confusing or muddled, steer clear. You will save yourself valuable time and money in the long run.

Be wary of titles other than those listed here. Where expertise is being claimed via a title (i.e. 'trauma-informed'), don't rely on that alone. Remember that almost anyone can give themselves any title they please in this arena. Probe. Check. Be curious. Ask them about their qualifications, training, experience, what they have written or researched on the subject. Be open-minded but sceptical.

Summing it up

No single type of therapist is better than another in every circumstance and with every person. Every psy-professional has their own area of expertise and ways of working. But ultimately, anyone properly trained and qualified and describing themselves by any of the job titles listed in this chapter should have a core set of skills that can help you. Most are well trained and keen to help. If they create an environment in which you feel safe to discuss your problems, and if you have confidence in them, irrespective of what they call themselves, you will likely join the vast majority of people who feel better off after having therapy.

The odds of having a good outcome will be greatly increased if you choose a treatment that has a sound evidence base, is matched to your particular circumstances and makes sense to you. So, our next chapter describes the different forms of therapy available and starts to guide you towards choosing which is most likely to be of help to you.

Ten things to remember

1. Do your research. How your therapist works and their level of competence are major factors in ensuring you get the help you need.
2. Don't waste money on expertise you don't need. If you don't need a specialism, don't pay for it.
3. Conversely, if you need someone with specialist skills in a particular area, make sure that's what you get.

4. Someone who really knows your profession or industry or understands your life circumstances might be more helpful, even if their length of training or professional status doesn't match that of others.
5. Most job titles in this area are not legally protected. Check that they are on one of the relevant statutory or accredited professional registers when you choose your therapist.
6. Don't be afraid to ask your therapist about their level of experience and training. If they are evasive or unclear, move on.
7. Don't make training and expertise the sole criteria for your choice. Interpersonal chemistry and fit really matter in therapy. If you don't get on with a therapist, they won't be able to help you.
8. There is no such thing as a perfect therapist, and you don't need the perfect therapist to make meaningful changes in your life.
9. Be vigilant when choosing a coach. Make sure you're happy with their level of training and professionalism and don't be seduced by exaggerated claims of overnight success.
10. Be wary of add-on titles suggesting a particular expertise. Probe and be curious. Be open-minded but sceptical.

Chapter 3
What's what?

Having got a handle on who's who, we are still left with the problem that there are currently more than 500 different forms of therapy from which to choose. Sure, one size doesn't fit all, but how do we make sense of so many different, competing treatments? But before you despair, most types of therapy can actually be grouped into a few main categories, which we'll consider below.

Therapy can be delivered in a few different ways and in different settings. Most therapy tends to involve a live therapist and client talking together in real time. However, since the Covid-19 pandemic, therapy is increasingly available online, as well as in person, and, but less often, via telephone. Some providers now also offer therapy via text, email, app and even chatbots – and we'll cover these more in Chapter 7 on technology.

As well as individual therapy, couples therapy – sometimes called 'couple counselling' or 'marriage guidance' – is becoming increasingly popular. This is also delivered online or in person. Group therapy too is offered online as well as in person, and is mostly available through the NHS and from some charities and private clinics. It doesn't suit everyone, but can be a useful way to get support from others in the same position as you, as well as helping you 'normalise' your feelings and realise that you're not alone. Family therapy, as the name implies, involves the whole family (or as many of the family members as are willing to be involved), with the aim of bringing to bear the resources of all those closely involved around the individual in stressful times – whether that's conflict between members (most often, parents and children) or the impact of one member's addiction or other mental health issue on the entire family.

Therapy is provided by the NHS, charities, private clinics or by individual therapists in private practice, working from their home or a rented room or office. There is no comprehensive research to suggest that any of these settings work better than others. Many employers also provide therapy for their staff. It is often short term and you won't have a great deal of choice about what you get.

The NHS also provides guided self-help therapy (NHS, 2022a). This is often your first offer if you refer yourself (or are referred by your GP) for NHS talking therapy. It generally involves following a workbook or online course, and is done on your own or with the support of a therapist. Then, if your problems still aren't resolved, you may get a limited number of therapy sessions one-to-one with a live therapist or, if you are really struggling, you may be referred to a psychologist or psychiatrist for assessment and treatment.

While therapy on the NHS is free, you are likely to face long waiting times before you see a therapist (Royal College of Psychiatrists, 2022). Therapy in private practice, by contrast, is usually readily available, but it is not free. The type of therapy you choose won't generally affect the cost, but the type of therapist you choose will – those who've trained for longer and who are more experienced usually charge more. Likewise, counsellors tend to charge less than psychotherapists, and private psychiatrists charge the most. Many, but not all, counsellors and psychotherapists offer a sliding scale, linked to their clients' income. Charities usually use a sliding scale too. Rates go out of date quickly, but for a rough indicator, one of the longest established charitable providers of therapy in London currently (2023 rates) charges £40 per session for those with an individual annual income of up to £35,000, and £80 for those with an income above £95,000. Even so, the organisation claims that these costs are up to 50% cheaper than the average private therapy session in London. Couples therapy tends to be more expensive than individual therapy, and executive coaching can be the most expensive of all.

So, with that context in place, let's now look at the main forms of therapy available to you, as you keep in mind your particular problem and ask yourself which is most likely to be helpful to you.

Cognitive behavioural therapy (CBT)

Cognitive behavioural therapy (CBT) is perhaps the best known and most widely available type of therapy. It helps you recognise how your thoughts, feelings and behaviour are all connected and influence each other. Simply put, the way we think or act in any situation makes a massive difference to how we feel about it.

Let's take an example. When a relationship ends, you can choose to learn from your mistakes, be grateful for the good times and perhaps realise your ex wasn't entirely right for you. You might take some time to lick your wounds. But you won't let this stop you talking to friends, continuing to socialise and, in time, looking to meet someone new.

If, instead, you think that the relationship ending means you are a failure, that nothing ever works out for you and that you always pick the wrong people, these thoughts will leave you feeling hopeless. That might well start to influence your behaviour and you may find yourself preferring to stay home when friends invite you out. Staying home will, in turn, leave you feeling lonely and unhappy. And it will also pretty much guarantee you won't meet somebody new.

In CBT, you learn how negative thoughts and behaviours affect you and what you can do to change them. You learn to recognise these 'automatic' and habitual thoughts and behaviours and can practise more helpful ways of responding. A CBT therapist will also often set you 'homework' tasks in between sessions. After all, therapy typically lasts for 50 minutes a week, but there are 167 other hours in those seven days that can be used to practise and hone new skills. Imagine learning a new language or musical instrument at the rate of just 50 minutes a week. The more you practise noticing and challenging your thoughts and trying out new behaviours, the better you get at it. It also means that, once your therapy is finished, you are able to use the tools yourself. This is partly why CBT tends to be quite a short-term form of therapy.

'Behavioural activation' is a particular type of CBT. It helps you recognise the link between what you do and your mood. Once you've established this link, you can plan practical changes in behaviour that are targeted at improving your mood. For example, you've stopped going out much and you don't much fancy going for a walk or meeting a friend for coffee, but you go anyway, knowing that you are likely to feel better afterwards and be glad that you did. As the name implies, behavioural activation does not directly target thoughts and feelings; it targets behaviours that improve the way you think and feel about life. It is often listed in the guidelines produced by the National Institute for Health and Care Excellence (NICE) for treatments offered in the NHS (see Chapter 1, and we cover this more in Chapter 4).

CBT is used in the NHS both for the more common problems like depression and anxiety and also for some of the more complex issues such as eating disorders, addictions, insomnia, phobias, post-traumatic stress disorder (PTSD) and obsessive-compulsive disorder. It is also used to help people cope with longstanding health problems, such as chronic pain and irritable bowel syndrome (IBS). CBT doesn't cure physical illnesses, of course, but it can help you cope better with the physical symptoms and lower your stress levels.

Whether CBT is right for you depends on your particular problem or issue. For example, therapy is often useful following a bereavement, and in this instance you might want space to explore what the person who has died meant to you, your feelings of loss and how you might begin to cope with everyday life again. But you are unlikely to need CBT techniques for this, as they are aimed at adjusting your way of thinking.

Acceptance and commitment therapy (ACT)

Acceptance and commitment therapy (ACT) has evolved from CBT to emphasise mindfulness and acceptance as key components of change. It views psychological distress as universal and normal. Therefore, it places the emphasis on accepting difficult things as an ordinary part of life, rather than trying to change them. ACT highlights how much energy we can spend trying to escape from, or control, events and experiences that are actually outside of our control.

Let's look at an example. You suffer from chronic back pain, despite having undergone surgery to ease it. You've been advised that daily exercise helps, even though it's hard to make time for it, and sometimes you resent having to do it. You could take the view that life is unfair and give up all hope of living the life you want, because of the pain. You could also spend a lot of time wishing the pain away and searching for cures and solutions online, and spend a lot of money on them. You could also spend the time you have with friends and family telling them about the detail and extent of your pain.

Instead, ACT suggests that you accept the pain as a regrettable fact of life and acknowledge that daily exercise helps. It emphasises the fact that, even though the pain stops you doing some things, there are many other things you can still do that are pleasurable. It also guides you to organise your life realistically and avoid trying to do too much on days when the pain is much worse, so you don't get angry, disappointed or surprised in those moments.

ACT is not trying to get you to look on the bright side or count your blessings; it is trying to get you to take a realistic view. Your therapist will help you step back and detach from your negative thoughts or your preoccupations about what life 'should' be like. You will also come to see that you have the ability to notice difficult thoughts and feelings and still choose how to respond. ACT tries to reconnect you with what is most important to you. This is the final part of ACT: you use the values you are committed to, not your passing thoughts and feelings, to guide your behaviour.

Dialectical behaviour therapy (DBT)

Dialectical behaviour therapy (DBT) is based on CBT, but it's adapted for people who feel especially intense emotions. For example, you might benefit from DBT if you experience extreme feelings of rejection, failure, isolation and a sense of victimisation. Or perhaps you feel devastation where sadness might usually be expected, or humiliation in place of disappointment, or furious rage instead of anger and annoyance. Those feelings might also lead to impulsive and harmful behaviours as you attempt to cope with them, such as substance abuse, speeding in your car, spending money you don't have, or self-harm and suicidal behaviour.

This type of therapy is more likely to work for you if you're committed to making positive changes and willing to take on challenges outside of the sessions. For example, you are likely to be asked to fill out a diary that tracks your emotions and actions and looks for patterns and triggers in your life, and to bring it to your next session. DBT teaches mindfulness skills that keep you focused on the present, enabling you to stay calm and not allow your emotions to spiral. Such skills allow you to recognise, label and accept intense emotions, without the need to react in an extreme or impulsive way. DBT also focuses on teaching you ways to communicate more effectively, such as listening to others, saying 'no' when you need to, and dealing with difficult people in an assertive way.

DBT is often available on the NHS. Although it was originally developed for a specific form of so-called personality disorder (borderline personality disorder, or BPD), some NHS services are also starting to offer DBT more widely, especially to young people. That said, accessing this type of therapy can be difficult as it isn't available everywhere and NHS waiting lists can be long. There is currently no official register of DBT therapists in the UK, but most internet directories let you filter your search by type of therapy.

Psychoanalysis

If brief problem-solving therapies, like CBT and ACT, are at one end of the spectrum, psychoanalysis is at the other. If you are in psychoanalysis, you will usually see your analyst several times a week, and analysis often continues for years. That's because psychoanalysis sees people as highly complex beings – far more complex than they first appear – and believes that our conscious mind is just the tip of the iceberg. So, given this complexity and that it has taken you a lifetime to become who you are, it follows that it will take considerable time and effort for you to understand how you came to be that way and to make choices to do things differently.

In psychoanalysis, you are encouraged to talk about whatever is on your mind, and, by and large, your psychoanalyst won't interrupt you. This is for the simple reason that they are giving you the opportunity to reveal what's happening at a less conscious level of your mind. They don't want to get in the way of that or interrupt your flow. In time, they will point out patterns, themes, contradictions, deeper meanings and connections in what you are saying. They will also notice what you might be trying to avoid talking about. They will do this in order to help you see how your less conscious thoughts may be affecting, or even dominating, your life.

Often the things that are hidden below the surface are those aspects that we don't want to admit about ourselves: our desire for money or status, our envy, our vanity, our aggression and our self-righteousness. Because they don't fit with our preferred view of ourselves, we try to keep them out of our consciousness.

Let's look at an example. Someone comes to therapy because of a difficult childhood. They describe their father as angry and demanding and their mother as heroic for putting up with him while also caring for the children and looking after the home. As well as talking about Dad, psychoanalysis would make space for more hidden feelings about Mum. Are there really only positive feelings towards her? Maybe Mum should have left the relationship? Or done more to ensure Dad didn't take his temper out on the kids? Maybe there is actually some anger towards her? Or maybe it's more like disappointment? Or disrespect? Maybe the client is determined not to get into the same sort of relationship themselves? Or maybe they are sworn off relationships altogether? Or maybe they assume that this is what women often have to put up with? Psychoanalysis would explore all of this, with the aim of transforming what is less conscious into something more conscious.

Although classical psychoanalysis is rare these days, lots of forms of therapy, especially psychoanalytic or psychodynamic psychotherapy, draw on the idea that we are influenced by things that we're not conscious of. While psychoanalysis is currently less popular, partly due to the expense and time commitment it involves, many of its ideas underpin today's discussions around the notion of free will and cognitive biases in decision-making.

Because of this frequency, duration and expense, psychoanalysis is not offered on the NHS. However, a short form of psychoanalytically informed therapy specifically designed for treating depression and anxiety – dynamic interpersonal therapy (DIT) – is available on the NHS and usually lasts between 16 and 20 sessions.

Counselling

Counselling is often used as a generic term for talking therapy and is sometimes used interchangeably with the terms 'therapy' or 'psychotherapy'. We are using it here in its classic sense to mean an approach to therapy that focuses on communicating non-judgemental warmth and genuineness and uses the skill of active, careful listening. This is often also known as person-centred, client-centred or non-directive counselling.

The assumption in counselling is that people have the potential to resolve their own problems and to grow in whatever direction they need. This will happen naturally if the counsellor demonstrates the core attributes of emotional warmth, empathy and genuineness and offers non-judgemental acceptance. If they do, then this is enough for the client to 'actualise' their own potential to grow, and they will do so as surely as plants and flowers grow in the right conditions.

The key principle guiding counselling is that the client is the expert in their own life and knows best what they need. Counselling therefore will not try to 'treat', advise, teach or lead you. Knowing that you will only change as and when you are ready, therapy of this sort will not try to direct you in any way. Counselling waits for you to be ready and will not push or prompt you to do things you don't want or find hard to do. Counselling also explicitly rejects the idea that the counsellor knows best and rejects the tools and techniques associated with most other forms of therapy that encourage you to do something differently. Instead, counselling relies on the fact that a deep sense of being understood and respected will, over time, create the conditions for you to change. The goal is less to solve issues or fix problems and more to help you grow to become who you 'truly are'.

Person-centred counselling of this sort works particularly well when people want to be heard and understood – perhaps when telling the story of your childhood for the first time. Bereavement counselling often takes this form too. Family members might want you to 'move on' or no longer feel comfortable with you expressing strong emotions of loss or sadness. In such situations, when you have no one else in your life capable of listening, counselling can be a lifeline.

Counselling is a disciplined, professional form of talking therapy, and not the same as befriending or mentorship, with which it is sometimes confused. It is a skilled process that depends on active, attentive listening while reflecting back accurately what has been said. It involves waiting patiently, paraphrasing and clarifying when necessary, and doing so without interrogating or jumping in with advice or reassurance. In other words, it offers the very things that are so often missing in everyday conversation with family and friends.

Interpersonal psychotherapy

Interpersonal psychotherapy is usually used as a short-term treatment for depression as it focuses on identifying how relationships are related to feelings of depression. It is based on the belief that, more than any other aspect of life, the quality of our relationships affects our mood. Interpersonal psychotherapy can be helpful for people who have difficult relationships or who are adjusting to transitions in their relationships or their roles, such as becoming a new parent, children leaving home, divorce or being made redundant.

Interpersonal psychotherapy was influenced by psychoanalysis and attachment theory, and also by CBT. Attachment theory is important to a number of the therapies described in this book, and especially to couples therapy, and is based on the idea that attachment is a biological and psychological necessity for survival. Decades of empirical research (Fraley, 2016) have shown that your earliest relationships are the most important in shaping how you act and what you expect in your relationships. Attachment science challenges the assumption that people tend to seek out those they think will make them happy in a relationship and that, instead, they tend to seek those who feel familiar.

Interpersonal psychotherapy is structured and time-limited (usually 12–16 weeks) but, unlike CBT, it makes no attempt to uncover distorted or 'dysfunctional' thoughts. Instead, the goal is to change relationship patterns. In this way, it draws on attachment theory in assuming that we function best when our needs for closeness and connection with others are met and that many mental health problems stem from our inability to make and keep good relationships.

Existential therapy

Existential therapy aims to deal with the big questions of life: isolation, death and the notion of meaninglessness. It recognises that human existence involves tragedy alongside the joys of life. It is more of an approach to therapy than a specific set of techniques. Existential therapy assumes that we are absolutely responsible for our choices. Outside forces impact us, but we always have the freedom to choose how to respond. An existential therapist will assume that often it is the failure to make those choices that keeps us stuck in life. Inaction is an action; indecision is a decision. So, your therapist will help you discover how you might be avoiding your freedom to choose and encourage you to risk using that freedom.

This type of therapy is likely to be useful when you are at a critical point in life that marks the passage from one stage to another: for example, coming to terms with middle age, coping with the breakdown of a marriage, adjusting to children leaving home, or dealing with the physical limitations of later life. It tends to work well for people who are at a crossroads or who are questioning the status quo. But it does also rely on you being able to find a therapist who is genuinely wise and capable of a wide-ranging understanding of what it means to live a good life.

It is unlikely to appeal to those who prefer a more practical approach. Existential therapy has tended to reject the idea that therapy can be measured and evaluated in quantitative ways, so if you are looking for a treatment that is strictly evidence-based, validated by robust trial data and focused on measurable outcomes, it's unlikely to appeal to you.

Integrative therapy

Many of the ideas within the different schools of therapy overlap and complement one another, and therapists frequently pick and choose across the various modalities to inform their approaches with clients. They describe this as 'integrative therapy'. In a 2023 survey of BACP members (BACP, 2023), who constitute the largest body of talking therapists in the UK, more than 40% identified themselves as offering 'integrative therapy', making it the most common type of therapy available outside the NHS (CBT is much more common within the NHS).

This idea of blending together several approaches to therapy has been shown to be useful. For example, emotion regulation skills can enhance the efficacy of CBT for people with depression (Kazantzis et al., 2018). But it is worth asking your therapist exactly what they are integrating, if that is not clear, as the term 'integrative' on its own doesn't mean very much. Simply put, you need to know what is being integrated before you know whether it is likely to suit you. You may also want to know which types of therapy your therapist has formally trained in and which ones they draw on most often.

Integrative therapy has become an increasingly popular way of providing a more tailored, personalised approach, as it recognises that different therapies are effective for different people (Boswell et al., 2010; Norcross & Wampold, 2018). But researchers also stress the need for integration to be based on the evidence of the component therapies' effectiveness (Norcross & Goldfried, 2019) and not simply on the preferences or interests of the therapist. So, again, you might want to ask your therapist about that, if it's important to you.

Couples therapy

There are different forms of couples therapy, depending on the way your therapist works – i.e. whether they apply a cognitive behavioural, problem-solving approach; whether they think in a more psychoanalytic way, or whether they use attachment theory, for example. Many will use a blend of approaches, and the best will often try to tailor this approach to you and your particular issue. As described below, most will tend to focus on how you communicate, resolve conflicts and manage the often strong emotions associated with being in a close relationship.

Some important research in this area suggests that emotions and how they are managed (or not) in a relationship are of most importance (Wiebe & Johnson, 2016). In simple terms, that means arguments are rarely *just* about what they seem to be about: coffee cups left by the dishwasher, who does the most housework or childcare, how clean your home should be, the importance of being on time, whose friends you see the most or who initiates sex. What you are really arguing about is not being seen or heard, understood or appreciated. Or maybe you are feeling controlled, spoken down to or belittled. Either way, the stuff of everyday life triggers intense feelings because they often have a bigger emotional meaning attached.

Couples therapy can help you think about how each of you expresses your emotions and how the inevitable conflicts that arise from being in a relationship are resolved. Often, one of the first things couples learn in therapy is that, to date, conflicts may never have genuinely been resolved and instead may have been ignored or brushed under the carpet. Or perhaps things just drifted back to normal with nothing being said, or maybe conflict was stored up and used as ammunition in future arguments. Couples therapy looks at what lies beneath your communication style, conflicts and complaints about one another.

Couples therapy also stresses the need to *manage* conflict constructively, because conflict is inevitable. Research suggests more than two thirds of arguments are about recurring problems, based in the differences between your personalities, preferences and how you each see the world (Fulwiler, 2012). Couples therapy therefore aims to help you accept these differences (and the strong feelings that go with them) while reducing your tendency to criticism, contempt, defensiveness or zoning out (Gottman, 2007) when disagreements arise. In therapy, you start to notice your own and your partner's patterns – your respective tendencies to attack, provoke, withdraw or silently sulk or seethe. You learn to discuss your preferences without criticising your partner, and to tackle conflict instead of letting it fester or spill over into contempt. You openly acknowledge your differences and, in time, you may even cherish your partner again in a way that you probably did when you first met.

A good couples therapist won't take sides but will help you see one another's perspective, even when one partner has behaved poorly or instigated an affair, for example. Therapy should enable you to feel sufficiently safe to open up and speak up and to explore your own and, in turn, your partner's experiences. Therapy will also focus on the strengths of the relationship – what is going right, your shared interests and responsibilities, the things you still admire and like about one another, as well as the reasons you fell in love in the first place.

Couples therapy will also usually talk about sex – who initiates it, how frequently it takes place, whether it is good or bad, and why it used to be so much better when you first met. Couples therapy generally takes the view that your sex life reflects what's going on in your relationship more generally (Crawley & Grant, 2007). Your therapist will usually introduce the topic early on, so you are not left worrying about if and when it's going to come up (Kerner, 2021).

The goal of couples therapy is less about 'fixing' the relationship or keeping you together and more about helping you work out what you each want and, if it turns out to be different, how you then cope with that. Sometimes, during the course of therapy, you may realise that your relationship has run its course – one person wants out, one is more invested than the other, or forgiveness is impossible after a betrayal. Even in such circumstances, you can use therapy to work out not just whether to separate but also how best to do so, especially when children, shared friends and finances are involved.

Family therapy

Family therapy does what it says on the tin: it provides therapy for the whole family – or as many as are willing and able to attend. It can be useful in any situation that causes stress or conflict within a family: behavioural problems in teens, parent–child conflicts, school refusal, illness or death in the family, caring for a family member with special needs, or the impact of substance abuse or other serious mental health issues.

Family therapy can help family members understand one another better, improve communication and learn skills to cope with difficult circumstances. It can help families identify the issues that contribute to conflict, pinpoint particular challenges, reflect on how they are handling them and learn to express emotions more productively. Of course, family therapy doesn't automatically solve problems like addiction or illness, but it can help family members spot unhelpful patterns, understand one another better, learn how to share thoughts and feelings openly and acquire skills to cope with the challenges of family life.

Let's say your son has depression. Quite likely, you and other family members are not sure how best to support him. Although everyone is concerned about his wellbeing, conversations with him, and between other family members, quickly end in disagreement and argument. Communication reduces as a result; perhaps the topic is avoided altogether and rifts in the family grow. Family therapy helps you acknowledge that you probably lack awareness about how best to help but it also considers whether sometimes families actively, if unintentionally, contribute to the problem. In the situation above, families learn how they can best be supportive and individual members reflect on their own behaviour, take seriously their own feelings of frustration about the situation and find better ways of managing it.

Family therapy encourages you to think about problems as belonging to the whole family, even when it is one individual experiencing the most pressing problem. Family therapy is concerned with the context in which the problem takes place. The basic idea is that, even if one person has a problem, the whole family has a significant role in maintaining the problem or making it better or worse.

This type of therapy is relatively rare outside of the NHS, where it tends to be used for families in crisis. But it is worth thinking about whether the pattern of family interactions cause or maintain the problem you are facing. Although the stereotype is that many children and teens are indifferent to, or embarrassed by, their family and their parents, this is far from the truth. Parents matter enormously to children of all ages. Good-quality interactions within a family provide support for all sorts of problems, just as poor-quality interactions make problems much worse for everyone involved.

Child psychotherapy/play therapy

Parents typically turn to child psychotherapy (or play therapy, depending on the age of the child) when they are concerned about their child's emotional development. Perhaps it's their ability to make friends, their refusal to attend school, bullying, 'fussy' eating, sleep patterns, soiling, anxiety or aggressive behaviour. Child psychotherapy can also help children deal with stressful life experiences such as a serious accident or chronic illness in the family. It is also helpful for much more commonplace events such as divorce, if children are struggling to cope with changes in the home or new custody arrangements.

With younger children, child psychotherapy usually takes the form of play therapy, for the simple reason that they lack the cognitive and verbal skills to express what they feel or explain what is troubling them. Although the feelings of young children are hard for them to express verbally, they can come out in play.

A play therapist will begin by listening to the parents' concerns and finding out a bit more about the child's history and any stresses in the family. They may also ask to talk to the school and any other significant adults in the child's life. They are likely to meet the parents at regular intervals to discuss progress in therapy, including any changes the parents have noticed at home. They will give the parents ideas on how to interact with their child and manage behaviour, but they won't discuss specific details from the sessions with the child. The parents' role is to get the child to the sessions on time, try out any new ways of interacting that are recommended and generally resist the urge to interfere too much. Therapy for children is private and confidential, just as it is for adults; it is up to them to share what goes on as, when and if they want to.

The therapist will have a selection of toys, craft materials, dressing-up props, board games and books. They will observe the child's interactions with the toys and games. Initially, they are looking to establish an atmosphere of safety. In time they are seeking to encourage the child to give full expression to their preferences and feelings. For some children, being in a busy home and classroom means that having the freedom to choose and their decisions respected may in itself be a first.

As the child grows more comfortable, more specific play activities will be introduced to target the issues the child is dealing with. Some child therapists will lead the child through guided activities to help them express themselves. For example, they might ask questions while the child draws, to try to gain insight into their thought process: who they drew first and why, what the animals in the picture might say to one another if they could speak, who lives in the house they have drawn. They might also play games with the child to encourage specific skills, such as turn-taking, problem-solving, the role of luck and how to cope with setbacks and defeat. They might start a story off and ask the child to come up with ideas for completing it. With some children, the challenge is to encourage them to fully express themselves; with others, it's about managing already overwhelming emotions.

With older children and those more able to vocalise their emotions, therapy will be a mix of play and talk, and it may be exclusively talk. The number of therapy sessions will depend on the needs of the individual child. Generally, child psychotherapy is a short-term intervention, but in some cases therapists work with children for several years. A child therapist may share information with other professionals (such as the child's school) for the benefit of the child, with their permission. They will also do this if they are concerned that a child is at risk of or being harmed or hurting others or themselves. Again, they will talk to the parents or carers about this first, where possible.

It is crucial that parents choose a qualified therapist for their child. There are several professional bodies to which child psychotherapists may belong. We strongly recommend that parents choose one whose register of members is accredited by the Professional Standards Authority.

Where autism, ADHD or other neurodevelopmental issues are suspected, the first port of call is the GP, who will guide parents or carers to resources appropriate to the age of the child and their particular issues. In some instances, the GP might recommend a specialist referral. A child psychotherapist might suggest a first-stage screening for neurodevelopmental issues, which they may be trained to administer and will then discuss with the parents/carers.

The problem with publicly funded child and adolescent mental health services is that the need far outweighs the resources available. The number of under-18s in contact with NHS mental health services in England rose by nearly 30% from 2020/21 to 2021/22 (NHS Digital, 2022a). The same survey (BBC News, 2022) indicated that mental disorder affects five children in every classroom (within the 7–16 age range). It prompted leading mental health charities to once again stress the need for urgent further investment, noting that the earlier a young person gets support for their mental health, the more effective that support is.

What about the other 490 types of therapy?

There are many other specific types of therapy, many with weird and wonderful names and acronyms: AEDP, ISDTP, CAT, biodynamic massage therapy, body psychotherapy, Human Givens, psychosynthesis, primal therapy, animal-assisted therapy, and more. The list is long. Many on that list have not been tested in robust trials.

But some types of therapy that sound no less odd, such as DIT (dynamic interpersonal therapy, as mentioned earlier), have been trialled and shown to be effective for particular problems, such as depression and/ or anxiety (Fonagy et al., 2020). As a consequence, DIT is available on the NHS, and has been for more than a decade. Others, such as REBT (rational emotive behaviour therapy) and CFT (compassion-focused therapy) are forms of CBT. Rational emotive behaviour therapy has five decades of research behind it (David et al., 2018), and compassion-focused therapy is now routinely available on the NHS, after recent research showed that, in 66% of relevant studies, it led to significant positive change (Craig et al., 2020).

Meanwhile, there are several well-known treatments with high profile advocates that actually have relatively little good quality evidence to support them. Many are not available in the NHS for this reason, or they are available in only very limited circumstances. We look at a few of them in more detail in Chapter 6.

In the end, the sheer number of different therapies available make this a complex and messy terrain to navigate. Realistically, no one can offer an assessment of 500 different types of therapy. But generally, you should be wary of brand names, jargon and fads. Therapy is prone to fads, just as medicine has been through the ages. Many of the current 'new kid on the block' therapies will go the same way as popular ideas from previous decades that now seem ridiculous – rebirthing, past life therapy and primal scream therapy, to name just a few.

Summing it up

As a rough guide, if a form of therapy is not available on the NHS, we suggest you think very carefully before deciding whether it is right for you. Generally, in healthcare, you want the treatment you receive to have been tried and tested, with published evidence that people have found it helpful, in their own accounts as well as in quantified research studies.

Therapy is a huge opportunity to change your life for the better. Don't pass this up for untrialled treatments that promise the earth. If it sounds too good to be true, it probably is. There are now more than four decades of evidence behind standard therapy techniques. They are not miracle cures. They do not work in all circumstances. But they do work, for most people, with most problems, most of the time.

However, you may have noticed there is a lot of common ground between therapies. All effective therapy works in a broadly similar way and is effective to about the same extent (Wampold, 2015). So, don't panic. If you are choosing a mainstream therapy that makes sense to you, and it is being delivered by a qualified therapist, then chances are it will help you. That's the case for more than 75% of people who have had therapy.

So, in the next chapter, we focus on how to get the right therapy for *you* – i.e. what treatment is likely to be the most effective for you and your particular problem.

Ten things to remember

1. Do your research. This chapter has outlined the main different types of therapy available to you; use it to guide what might work for your particular problem.
2. Although there are 500 different types of therapy, don't despair. Most fall into the 10 main categories we've described in this chapter.
3. Don't assume all therapy is the same. Psychoanalysis and CBT, for example, focus on different things and both will feel very different to the client.
4. A mainstream therapy that fits your problem and is supported by the evidence is likely to result in you being able to make meaningful changes in your life.
5. If a type of therapy is not available on the NHS or is only available in very limited circumstances, think carefully about whether it is right for you.
6. There are several well-known treatments with high profile advocates that actually have relatively little good quality evidence to support them.
7. There are now more than four decades of evidence behind standard therapy techniques. For most people, with most problems, most of the time, those therapies work.
8. Generally, you should be wary of fads. Therapy is prone to them, just as medicine has been through the ages.

9. Although we've been distinguishing between different types of therapy, there is a lot of common ground between them. Many researchers suggest that all effective therapy works in a similar way and is effective to about the same extent.
10. Don't panic. If you are choosing a mainstream therapy that makes sense to you and is delivered by a qualified therapist, then the chances are it will help you. That's the case for more than 75% of people who have had therapy.

Chapter 4
Your preferences and what will work for you

Obsessive and compulsive thoughts, heartbreak after an affair, being stuck in a deep depression or your teenage child refusing school are all very real problems. But they are also very different. In this chapter, we look at which type of therapy works best for which type of problem. We also look at what is likely to work best for you. Your choice of therapy needs to align with your personality and the way you think about the world; otherwise, it's unlikely you'll stick with it or get much from it. If you're a deeply practical person who likes tools and solutions, you'll prefer a different kind of therapy to someone who wants to take time to understand how you ended up where you are.

You might expect there to be one type of therapy that is better for a particular problem, but in fact many different types of therapy have been shown to be helpful and no one single type of therapy has been proven to work for everyone and for every problem (Layard & Clark, 2015a). Cognitive behavioural therapy (CBT) is recommended most often by the National Institute for Health and Care Excellence (NICE), the independent body that produces guidelines for treatments that can be offered on the NHS, but so too are several other forms of therapy that have also been shown to be effective for the same common mental health problems. For example, the NICE guidelines for mild to moderate depression recommend several forms of therapy.

That means you often have a choice, especially if you are paying for therapy privately. If two or more treatments work pretty much the same on average, then in theory you could pick either or any of them. But in practice, your choice of therapy needs to align with your preferences and how you make sense of the world. So, that's where we'll start, by looking at what type of therapy makes most sense to you. We'll then consider what the research evidence says about what works for your particular problem.

What suits you – your personality and preferences

If you want therapy to keep you focused on a specific issue and challenge your ways of thinking, then CBT and practical problem-solving approaches might suit you best. But if you believe that much of what you do is unconscious, influenced by your childhood experiences and upbringing, and you'd like the space to explore that, then you might find a psychoanalytic approach more helpful.

If you struggle in relationships, you might want to work with a therapist who puts attachment theory at the heart of how they try to help. Similarly, if you're looking to talk about difficult events in your life with someone who will listen in a warm, non-judgemental way while you find your own way forward, then person-centred counselling might work best.

These are important considerations that are not just about what you are likely to prefer; they will also influence the outcomes you'll get from therapy. Numerous studies show that therapy that matches clients' preferences is associated with more positive outcomes (Cooper et al., 2017). Clients have a 58% chance of greater improvement and are about half as likely to drop out if they get their choice of therapy than if they don't (Swift & Callahan, 2009a). We also know that therapy is much more likely to be effective if you have confidence in it (Devilly & Borkovec, 2000) and you expect it to work (this is true of medical treatments too). After all, you are unlikely to fully engage with an approach you don't buy into, and you may ultimately even stop going altogether.

So, consider the questions below and use them to help you think about which approach to therapy makes most sense to you. The questions are drawn from a well-researched checklist (Cooper & Norcross, 2015), the Cooper-Norcross Inventory of Preferences (C-NIP), that was developed to help people explore their therapy preferences. Spend some time thinking about the questions. It will pay off. You are not just choosing something you prefer; you're increasing the odds of getting the best possible outcome from a considerable investment of time and money.

If you find the prompts useful, you can go online and do the full 18-item assessment (Cooper & Norcross, 2019).[1]

1. Do you have a strong preference to focus on goals and for therapy to have structure, to teach coping skills and include tasks to complete outside the session? Do you want to be led by your therapist or do you want them to follow your lead?

CBT (along with DBT and ACT, which are forms of CBT) is most likely to provide structure and focus. Person-centred counselling and psychoanalysis are probably the least likely to do so. How structured other forms of therapy are will depend on the style of the therapist – some couples, family and child therapists will be quite directive during sessions and will provide suggestions for reading or suggest tasks outside of your sessions. Others won't. If you have clear preferences, it's always best to let your therapist know and ask them how they work. Generally, shorter-term therapy will be more goal focused.

2. Do you want to focus mainly on thoughts or feelings? Would you be comfortable talking about the therapy relationship itself? For example, do you recognise that your patterns of thinking and behaviour will show up in therapy too? Would you like to be encouraged to express strong feelings or would you find that uncomfortable and prefer not to do so?

DIT will focus on your feelings and also what's going on between you and your therapist during the session. Other psychoanalytic forms of therapy will do the same. CBT is much less likely to do this. Counselling is also less likely to do so unless you raise it. However, counselling will encourage you to experience any strong feelings and put them into words. CBT will focus instead on thoughts and behaviour as the way to change your emotions and will not generally encourage you to express strong feelings for their own sake. Counselling is less likely to challenge so-called distorted or

1. See https://pluralisticpractice.com/wp-content/uploads/2019/06/C-NIP1.1-2019-04-04-with-guidelines.pdf

dysfunctional thoughts, but CBT will specifically and frequently do so. In psychoanalysis, your therapist will notice patterns in your thinking style and may point them out to you, but they won't suggest how to restructure them in the way that CBT would.

3. Would it be helpful to reflect on your childhood and upbringing, or would you prefer to focus on life in the present?

Attachment-based approaches in particular will focus on your early years and how those first relationship patterns continue to show up and influence your relationships today. Interpersonal psychotherapy (which draws on attachment theory) will focus on the quality of your relationships and particularly how they affect your mood, but will tend to do so more in the present. DIT will do a mix of both. CBT will not make your childhood the focus of therapy to the same extent, although don't assume that CBT never looks at your past – it will in certain circumstances and if it is important to you. Counselling will be led almost entirely by what you choose to focus on.

4. Would you like your therapist to confront your behaviour if they think it is causing problems for you? Or would you prefer them to be supportive at all times? Similarly, should they interrupt you if you've strayed from the point, or would you find that disrespectful?

CBT therapists in the main are more likely to challenge you to do things differently, especially outside of sessions (for example, to speak up at work or ask someone out on a date). CBT will use the focus agreed with you at the start of therapy to bring you back to the point if you deviate too much. Shorter-term types of therapy like DIT and interpersonal psychotherapy will similarly use the focus you have agreed to help keep you on track, but they won't challenge your thinking in the way CBT will. Psychoanalysis specifically encourages you to follow where your mind goes, in order to pick up what is going on at a less conscious level; it will certainly not interrupt you if you've strayed from any supposed point. Most forms of open-ended counselling will not do so either. Psychoanalysis may well interpret the behaviour you are talking about as having an underlying or less conscious meaning, but in contrast to CBT, it will not try to alter this or make suggestions for behaving differently. Person-centred counselling might point out some of the ways you cause problems for yourself but would leave it up to you to decide if and how you want to change that.

While your answers to these questions do not automatically or simply translate into a particular type of therapy, hopefully you can begin to see that they often point you in a particular direction. For example, the amount of challenge and guidance you want will lead you towards or away from CBT (including ACT and DBT). Similarly, if you are not so interested in working with a specific focus and you would prefer to be predominantly supported rather than challenged by your therapist, you might prefer person-centred counselling. And if you want to explore your early childhood and are curious about how your patterns of relating to people show up in therapy, then you might prefer a more psychoanalytic approach, and perhaps one that draws on attachment theory in particular.

Short-term therapy will necessarily have more focus and structure than open-ended approaches. For some people, the value of therapy, especially when it's paid for privately, is that there is no rush; you can say whatever you want, in the way you want, at the pace that you want. For others, the point is to solve problems and do so as quickly as possible – you are conscious of cost, you want tools and techniques you can take away, and you get lost in your own thoughts if you're not given structure and guidance.

Where therapists are integrating different approaches, you need to think even more carefully about what that might mean for you and whether it will suit you.

Where you are not completely sure about what is being offered, the simplest thing to do is to ask your prospective therapist to explain how they work. Any decent therapist will be only too happy to describe that to you in simple terms. And if they can't or won't, move on, continue the search, find someone who can.

Finally, remember that, while you'll likely want a mix of support *and* challenge, you will have a natural tendency to prefer one more than the other. So try to get in touch with your preferences. Be honest. Take your instincts seriously. You probably know what will work best for you. Therapy is hard. It requires you to be honest about difficult thoughts and feelings. You won't always want to show up for your sessions and you won't always enjoy them. It's a lot like the gym in that respect. But you'll be much more likely to persevere and get more out of it if you believe in the approach you've chosen.

So, keep your preferences in mind as you go on to read about the evidence for what type of therapy works best for particular types of problems, which we will discuss later in this chapter.

How good is the evidence?

Tuning into your preferences will help you choose the right type of therapy, but you also need to consider what the research says works best for your particular type of problem.

There has been a dramatic shift in emphasis to evidence-based practice, rather than just professional opinion, in all forms of healthcare over the past few decades. In the UK, this has been most visible in the form of the guidelines issued by NICE. As we've previously explained, NICE is the independent body that is charged by the UK government with reviewing and recommending the most clinically effective (and cost-effective) treatments for use in our public health (NHS) and social care services. NICE exists to make sure taxpayers' money is spent wisely on the most effective treatments in all areas of health and social care, including mental health. Its recommendations have become so influential that NICE now has a growing international role too, sharing its recommendations with other countries to drive improvements in their health and social care systems.

For each mental health condition, NICE convenes a committee drawn from expert clinicians, researchers and patients/users. Drawing on the latest research, the committee agrees the treatments to recommend on the basis of the research evidence for their clinical and cost effectiveness. The process is intended to be independent of government and lobbying, although, as you'll see, there is disagreement about exactly what the terms 'clinical effectiveness' and 'cost effectiveness' mean and how best to define them.

In the area of mental health, NICE sets the guidelines for the NHS in terms of which types of therapy it should provide and which psychiatric medications are helpful (we cover medication in more detail in Chapter 8). In order to do so, it draws on evidence from randomised control trials (RCTs) in particular. RCTs randomly assign a group of patients with the same condition into two groups; one group receives the treatment, and the other group (the control) doesn't (sometimes they are given something called a placebo – an identical treatment that is inert and will have no therapeutic effect). The outcomes for the two groups are then compared, and any variables (external influences) ruled out. The differences between the two groups in terms of outcome can then be seen as the result of the intervention used and not chance or any other external factor.

For those reasons, RCTs are often described as the gold standard for evidence (Hariton & Locascio, 2018) and are now the universal means of assessing which treatments work best in medicine and healthcare, whether that's a new drug, different forms of cancer surgery or a type of therapy (Layard & Clark, 2015a). RCTs often show us things that we wouldn't otherwise have known – perhaps the most dramatic example being the trial that ended 100 years of radical mastectomies for breast cancer. The study (Fisher et al., 1981) showed that half a million women who had mutilating operations could have had equally good outcomes with a simple lumpectomy – the opposite of what many experts thought at the time. Similar trials have been done on interventions such as providing psychological debriefing to survivors very soon after a traumatic event or accident. Research (Mayou et al., 2000) showed that what seems like a humane and common-sense intervention is actually unhelpful and slows down natural recovery.

It's clear from experiments like these that we need carefully controlled scientific trials in healthcare, medicine and public life more generally to show us what works and what doesn't. The truth is, subject matter experts often get it wrong. Doctors, clinicians and professionals are nowhere near as smart as they think they are (Navasky & Cerf, 1998). That includes therapists. Judgement based not on hard data but on clinical experience often turns out to be mistaken (Redelmeier et al., 2001). Sometimes dangerously so. The history of medicine is littered with eminent people who thought they knew best but who were in fact seriously harming, and sometimes killing, their patients (Dimidjian, 2019).

What about other forms of evidence?

While relatively few scientists are critical of RCTs, many do point out their limits and the limitations of relying on only one form of evidence. NICE has been criticised (Moncrieff & Timimi, 2013) for allowing RCTs to become the primary, if not only, measure of effectiveness and for not acknowledging other forms of evidence, such as case studies, interviews and observations. The complaint is that, while large-scale quantitative studies might be appropriate for medical research, psychological distress is very different and is often better measured by qualitative methods that observe and describe, rather than statistical analysis. For example, if you go to therapy seeking more meaning in your life, to grow as a person or to understand more about yourself, it's hard to quantify whether therapy has helped and by how much and to rule out multiple other factors in your life that might also contribute to your improved mood. It's easier to do that for shorter therapies that follow a strict protocol and target very specific symptoms, such as those of a phobia.

There are methodological problems with RCTs too: high drop-out rates (if participants drop out of a trial, they tend not be included in the final statistical analyses); difficulties in creating a truly comparable control group (if a placebo is being used, the control group must not know that they are getting a fake intervention), and potential conflicts of interest among the researchers, peer reviewers and the journals that publish the studies (these days, researchers generally have to declare potential conflicts of interest in any journal articles, but it may not always happen) (Shedler, 2018)). As we describe in Chapter 8, these criticisms are particularly relevant in the contemporary debate about whether psychiatric medication and psychedelic-assisted therapy can be helpful in improving mental health.

NICE has also been criticised (Watson, 2019) for using a research method that relies on diagnosis for its recommendations about which type of therapy works best, when many types of therapy, such as counselling, reject the very notion of mental disorders, diagnosis and treatment (Sanders & Tolan, 2023). Until 2021, there had never been a randomised controlled trial of counselling for depression, for example (Barkham et al., 2021a). So, because a type of therapy needs a positive finding from RCTs to be included in NICE guidelines, counselling has struggled to get recognition. As a consequence, counselling is not widely offered in NHS Talking Therapies services in England. This doesn't mean that counselling won't help you; it just means there is far less evidence from RCTs (barely any) that it will.

Legitimate concerns around the application of RCTs to psychotherapy are acknowledged even by those who advocate their use (Lemma et al., 2011). Perhaps the most obvious and repeated criticism (Ernest et al., 2015) is that the people recruited in clinical trials often have no co-occurring or overlapping conditions (very different from what tends to be the case in real life, where people often have multiple mental health problems). Consequently, the conclusions from these trials only truly apply to a limited group who are being treated in 'laboratory' conditions. Also, while RCTs are good at predicting averages, they do not tell us why some interventions work better for some people and not others, and so mask individual and sub-group differences (Deaton & Cartwright, 2016). Finally, RCTs are expensive (because they need large numbers of participants to achieve statistical significance), meaning only the types of therapy likely to be of interest to universities or hospitals or useful to pharmaceutical companies developing new products tend to be trialled.

This is not to say that RCTs shouldn't be used, but rather that, if qualitative research methods were added to the mix, it would create a richer picture. Epidemiological data, clinical observations and single-case experiments all go to create a better-rounded approach. Given RCTs are not the only scientifically valid evaluation method (Clay, 2010), and no one research design is perfect, integrating multiple sources of data should, arguably, be the norm. Those who argue that no one type of research should have a monopoly on the truth also point out that, of Galileo, Darwin, Einstein, Marie Curie and Stephen Hawking, not one of them ever conducted an RCT (Shedler, 2017).

In the end, even those who express concerns about RCTs (see, for example, Sanders et al., 2021) acknowledge that we now live in an evidence-driven world. RCTs have been used for more than 70 years to compare the effectiveness of new medicines (Haynes et al., 2012), and they were central to the roll-out of the Covid vaccines (Hallas et al., 2021). Advocates for RCTs (Lilienfeld et al., 2018) are clear that they are neither perfect nor a 'gold standard', but even with those limitations in mind, they say we should continue to assign greater weight to well-conducted RCTs than to other types of research when choosing what kind of therapy we have. That's the stance that NICE takes, and their recommendations and guidelines shape how NHS mental health budgets are spent.

So, what does NICE recommend?

With that in mind, what does NICE recommend, particularly, for the two most common mental health conditions affecting adults in the UK – depression and anxiety?

It's important to remember that these are the treatments for which NICE considers *there is sufficient and sufficiently robust evidence* of their effectiveness. NICE recommendations influence what services you'll get offered via the NHS; if you go private, you will have access to all the various therapies that you can find offered by therapists listed on the main online directories. NICE approval is undoubtedly a useful guide for the general public as to which therapies can be expected to be helpful – a kite mark of quality, if you like – but not all available therapies will have been researched to the same depth and rigour, just because they don't attract research funding, so they won't feature on the NICE lists.

Depression

NICE recommends (2022) 'stepped care' or 'matched care' for depression. This means you will be offered psychological treatment at the level of intensity your symptoms merit. So, with milder to moderate depression, you will start under the care of a practitioner who probably isn't a qualified counsellor but will have some training in CBT techniques following, in many cases, a psychology degree. This is a 'low-intensity' intervention, in NHS speak. At that level of depression, NICE recommends as your first-line treatment (in descending order of clinical and cost effectiveness) guided self-help, group CBT, group behavioural activation, individual CBT or behavioural activation, group exercise, group mindfulness or meditation, interpersonal psychotherapy, a course of an SSRI antidepressant, counselling or short-term psychodynamic psychotherapy.

Randomised control trials of self-help versions of cognitive behaviour therapy delivered online, via a computer programme or through an app, have shown benefits for mild to moderate depression, bulimia and many anxiety disorders (Layard & Clark,

2015a). In most cases, though, success rates were even better when the self-help was guided by a health professional providing regular, brief support via telephone, email or text message. NICE has therefore recently added a limited number of apps and online programmes to its recommendations for treatment of depression and anxiety, but with the proviso that they should be used alongside support from a trained practitioner (NICE, 2023).

If you have more severe depression, you will be 'stepped up' to see a 'high-intensity' therapist for one-to-one sessions and your first-line treatment options could include (again in the same descending order of clinical and cost-effectiveness) individual CBT with an antidepressant, individual CBT, individual behavioural activation, an antidepressant from a wider range of types, individual problem-solving, counselling, short-term psychodynamic psychotherapy, interpersonal psychotherapy, guided self-help or group exercise.

NICE also recommends behavioural couples therapy for people with depression where relationship problems could be contributing to their symptoms and involving their partner might help in treating their depression.

At all stages, NICE recommends that the practitioner discusses the options available with you and matches what you choose to your needs and preferences. If you ask for something that has worked for you before, they should try to provide that again, so long as they think it will be effective.

If these treatments haven't produced any benefits after four weeks of antidepressant medication or four to six weeks of psychological treatment or combined medication and therapy treatment, the recommended approach is to look at your personal and social life and explore with the therapist the factors that might be causing your depression and address them, or look to see if there could be a health condition in the mix, and then try other methods (increasing or switching your medication, for example, or offering more intense psychotherapy).

If these don't help, you may be referred to see a psychologist and possibly a psychiatrist.

Anxiety

For generalised anxiety disorder (GAD), NICE recommends

CBT-based self-help and psychoeducation (or guided self-help) as the initial lower-intensity intervention, escalating to individual CBT as a high-intensity intervention if needed. Treatment with medication can be considered if you haven't responded to earlier interventions, or if you are at high risk of self-harm.

For mild to moderate panic disorder, individual self-help or guided self-help is recommended. If you suffer with moderate to severe panic disorder, the guidance is to consider CBT or antidepressants if the problem is longstanding or if you haven't benefitted from therapy (or if you declined it). If you've tried two of these interventions and still have significant symptoms, the guidance suggests referral to specialist mental health services.

Individual or group CBT, including exposure and response prevention (ERP), should be offered if you suffer from mild to moderate obsessive compulsive disorder (OCD). People who have moderate or severe functional impairment or have another common mental health problem alongside OCD should be offered CBT (including ERP) or antidepressant medication. If you have long-standing OCD or severe and disabling symptoms, then referral to a specialist mental health service is likely to be considered. This should also be offered if you have not benefitted from two courses of CBT combined with antidepressant medication.

For post-traumatic stress disorder, NICE recommends CBT, or eye movement desensitisation reprocessing therapy (EMDR) in more limited circumstances (many experts (Layard & Clark, 2015a) consider EMDR to be a form of CBT). Drug treatment should only be offered if you decline therapy or express a preference for drug treatment.

NICE recommends individual CBT for social anxiety disorder. If you don't want CBT, then a drug treatment can be offered. If you decline CBT and drug treatment, then short-term psychodynamic therapy can be offered, but it is less clinically effective.

Other mental health issues

NICE also makes recommendations for less common mental health problems, such as eating disorders, personality disorders and substance dependence. For bulimia, they recommend CBT and interpersonal psychotherapy. For anorexia, they recommend

CBT, interpersonal psychotherapy, cognitive analytic therapy (CAT) and an inpatient weight-gain programme if you are dangerously underweight. For schizophrenia, it recommends CBT and family therapy.

NICE does not currently recommend a particular treatment for borderline personality disorder but it does list some approaches that have been shown to be better than standard care or other interventions in at least one randomised control trial. They include schema-focused cognitive therapy, mentalization-based therapy and dialectical behavioural therapy.

For antisocial personality disorder, group-based CBT is recommended; for alcohol dependence, motivational interviewing, behavioural couples therapy and CBT are recommended; for drug dependence, it's motivational interviewing, contingency management (incentives for abstinence, contingent on negative urine test etc.), behavioural couples therapy (only where the partner doesn't use drugs) and evidence-based psychological therapy (i.e. the approaches listed above for depression and anxiety).

Last, NICE recommends psychological therapy for physical conditions such as irritable bowel syndrome, chronic pain and chronic fatigue. That doesn't mean those conditions are 'all in the mind'; rather, it is welcome acknowledgement, where it often wasn't acknowledged before, that there is a link between mind and body and that changing how you think about your pain can help you cope with it much better.

Again, you need to check the NICE online guidance for specific recommendations. Bear in mind that it carries out periodic reviews of the evidence, to take account of new treatments and new research, and the recommendations may then be updated.

Also note that for young people, the guidance for high and low intensity treatments for each problem is different from that for adults. And, while many treatment options overlap, they do also vary and you should check the latest guidelines online and discuss the options with your GP if you are seeking treatment via the NHS.

Horses for courses?

Due to the number of RCTs into CBT, which is more easily researched using quantitative methods than most other talking therapies, NICE guidelines tend to favour CBT. For example, person-centred counselling is mostly included in the NHS Talking Therapies offer as a second option primarily because of the lack of RCTs to support its effectiveness (Barkham et al., 2021a).

So, while there are good reasons for considering CBT for many problems, it is not superior to all other types of therapy, except for anxiety disorders. Reaching for the NICE guidelines won't always be your best starting point: they are dense and sometimes difficult to make sense of (although these days much more effort is made to simplify them for the general public). But they do offer a good overview of the current state of the evidence about what works for your particular problem.

Indeed, as previously stated, not only is no one type of therapy right in every instance but many head-to-head comparisons of different types of therapy indicate broadly similar effects (Luborsky et al., 2002). An important large-scale comparison of CBT with other treatments for depression found similar results from them all (Cuijpers et al., 2013). These findings have led some to take the view that, because various therapies work for common conditions and because different therapies work for different conditions, it follows that all therapy works about the same (Lilienfeld & Arkowitz, 2012). Some therapists repeat this claim to clients. But it's not quite right.

The research most associated with the idea that all therapy works to the same extent is clear that some types of therapy *are* more effective than others (Fonagy & Wampold, cited in Schizofrenidagene, 2016). So too is a book considered the 'bible' in this field, *Evidence-based Psychotherapy Relationships* (Norcross & Lambert, 2019). Its authors conclude that particular treatment methods do make a difference, especially in more complex or severe cases, but the jury remains out on precisely by how much.

And this is where NICE comes in. It tries to reconcile genuine, ongoing disagreements among researchers. For example, the idea that CBT works best for anxiety disorders was disputed by some of the most prominent researchers in psychotherapy more than a decade ago (Benish et al., 2008). They found evidence to suggest that all the types of therapy they compared worked about the same (for PTSD, in particular). Three years later, other well-respected researchers refuted those findings (Ehlers et al., 2010). That's frustrating if you want to know what the best treatment is, but that's how science works. NICE keeps up with the evidence and exercises a judgement on what is currently available – albeit a flawed one, or an imperfect one, or a perfectly sensible one, depending on your point of view.

To sum up, research shows that there is no one-size-fits-all approach to treating mental health issues (Layard & Clark, 2015a). But it also shows that particular treatment methods for particular problems do still matter. NICE makes specific recommendations for specific conditions predominantly on the basis of large-scale quantitative trials. Relying mostly on that type of evidence may strike you as essential for scientific progress (Lilienfeld et al., 2018), or as a reason to be deeply sceptical of those types of guidelines (Shedler, 2017).

There are still many instances where NICE makes no recommendations at all: relationship problems and feeling 'stuck', for example, which are arguably some of the most common reasons why people come to therapy. And of course, NICE is not the only source of information. In the private sector, you are completely free to ignore its recommendations. As is your therapist. If you are interested in other points of view, many mental health charity websites have useful information about therapy, often including first person accounts – we list some of the best in the 'Further Reading and Resources' section at the end of this book. The main professional membership bodies also have useful information for clients, as do the main directory listing sites, such as the Welldoing and Counselling directories.[2,3] Together they offer a mix of blogs, videos, animations and brief overviews of different treatment types that can all help you think through and choose the therapy that's right for you.

Final reflections to guide your choice

Before we sum up the complex terrain we have covered in this chapter, we offer some reflections below, to help you hone in on what type of therapy is right for you. As you read the prompts, think about what resonates with you and challenge yourself to match them to a therapy we have described in this chapter.

2. https://welldoing.org

3. https://www.counselling-directory.org.uk

- ***Too much focus on the past can overlook the importance of the present***

Short-term, practical problem-solving therapies with a present-day focus can be highly effective in helping you with immediate, pressing problems. If you can't get up to give the kids breakfast and take them to school because of severe depression, you need the quickest fix available. If you're in a hole, you need a way to get out first, before you need a detailed understanding of how you got there. Plus, there is often surprisingly little relationship between the cause of the problem and the solution to it (de Shazer, 1985) and talking about the pain of your past may have next to no impact on how to solve problems in the present. In goal-driven, short-term, solution-focused approaches, the problems of the past are sometimes best seen as just 'damn bad luck' (de Shazer, 1985) and the way to build change is simply to do more of what already works.

- ***Too much focus on the present can overlook the importance of the past***

Your early years have an enormous influence on how your brain has developed. Early disadvantage, neglect and abuse set you up for heightened vulnerability to mental distress (Gilbert, 2009). Generally, short-term problem-solving therapy will not focus on your past, meaning that the question of why you are the way you are and why you keep repeating the same mistakes goes unanswered. Longer-term, open-ended therapy assumes you have been impacted by the events of your past and that your current difficulties do not arise in vacuum. Knowing why you act a certain way won't solve your problem on its own, but it can free you from the sense that something is wrong with you. Therapy that focuses on the past sheds light on your current difficulties and how to resolve destructive habits that otherwise keep repeating.

- ***Therapy isn't just about fixing problems, it's about support and growth too***

While fixing problems is important, therapy can also be thought of as 'having someone in your corner' – someone to help you be the best possible emotional version of yourself. In this respect, therapy is similar to the way you might work with a personal trainer to build fitness or recover from injury. Elite athletes have coaches, not because they aren't good at what they do but because they want to keep developing or sustain peak performance over long periods of time. Therapy works in the same way – it's about growth, improvement and sustaining gains, not just solving problems or fixing what isn't working.

- ***Sometimes you need time to make sense of your problems***

Short-term therapy, even when it's the best option for the specific problem you are facing, may not suit your temperament – perhaps you need time and space to make sense of your difficulties. While the better therapists will adjust the pace of the CBT to suit you (Beck, 2005), some shorter-term treatments don't leave much space for building trust, which is often essential before you can share past hurts. You may need to feel confident you will be heard and understood before you tell someone your inner secrets and distress. At other times, you might know something is wrong, but you might not know exactly what it is. Maybe you've got a number of issues. Maybe you feel anxious *and* depressed. Maybe you fear your career is going nowhere or that your partner no longer loves you. Maybe you've also got compulsive habits around food or drink. In this case, you might need space to notice the multiple problems and to work out what's most important. Short-term problem-solving therapy can be helpful in providing a focus and breaking problems down into manageable challenges, but it may not offer you the breathing space needed to really work out what's most important to you.

- ***Sometimes you need time to stop and listen to yourself***

Life is frantic. Therapy isn't just another place to go to take action or do work. It can also be a place of asylum and respite. A place to catch your breath and change pace. A moment in the week to drop the game face and reflect deeply. A place to sit back and hear yourself think. Forms of therapy that focus on listening deeply (counselling and psychoanalysis) can provide this. Sometimes you'll be surprised by your thoughts in therapy – by what you hear yourself saying or find yourself thinking. You might realise that something was more important to you than you first thought, or that you are actually less bothered about a stressful situation at work than you initially supposed. Types of therapy that help you find a sharp focus and set clear goals can be useful, but if they move into that stage too soon, they can rob you of the space to think and reflect.

- ***Some problems take time to resolve (irrespective of your preferences)***

One of the most obvious reasons why people favour therapy like CBT is because it is thought to be quick and practical. According to the research, that's true for the more common mental health problems – between eight to 16 sessions, in the case of depression (NICE, 2022), depending on severity. But it's not the case for complex issues like psychosis or eating disorders. The guidelines for adults suffering from anorexia (NICE, 2017), for example, suggest up to 40 CBT sessions over 40 weeks, with twice-weekly sessions in the first two to three weeks. That's an intense, time-consuming treatment lasting a year or so. So, if you have a complex issue like an eating disorder, addiction or psychosis, whatever type of therapy you choose, it will take longer to treat.

- ***Therapy is somewhere to say the unsayable***

Therapy is a place to say what's on your mind – no pretences, no need to put on a brave face or spare anyone's feelings. You can wonder if you're in the right relationship or confess how boring you find family life or that you hate your job and envy your friends. You can think about what would have happened if you'd married so-and-so, got the promotion you missed out on, or how people will remember you when you die – such questions tend to get crowded out by daily life and are hard to talk about even with friends. Generally shorter-term, problem-solving therapies are less geared up for this. In more open-ended, psychoanalytic or existential approaches, your therapist might also point out what's not being said, reminding you that everything is on the table, even the things you dread, hate, are ashamed of or long for. The aim of therapy, from this perspective, is not to alleviate symptoms of distress but to help you get to know yourself as fully as possible and to accept and embrace who you are.

- ***Therapy is somewhere your therapist can say the unsayable***

Sometimes you can go round in circles in therapy, rehearsing the same disappointments, difficulties and dilemmas, and sometimes you need to be confronted with that fact. Of course, that needs to be done respectfully, but often it is best done directly. Are you willing to make a change? Do you recognise your role in your problems? Therapy isn't just about sympathy and a listening ear. Your therapist might need to say the unsayable: are your husband, kids, neighbours or boss really all so disappointing or rude, or do you play a role too? Your partner cheated on you, but what was happening in the relationship before that point and how might that have contributed? A safe and confidential space is all well and good, but it is often not enough to generate change on its own. For that, you need challenge too. Therapy is not somewhere to hide out as the victim of life. Therapy aims to bring about what is best for you; it does not accept that the mess you are currently in is the best you can do.

- ***Making sense of relationship problems usually means your partner needs to be there too***

Individual therapy can help you with relationship issues but sometimes you need to work on the problems together with your partner. Cognitive-behavioural couple therapy, integrative behavioural couple therapy, and emotionally focused couple therapy (Wiebe & Johnson, 2016) all have sufficient evidence to be considered well-established treatments for relationship distress (Lebow & Snyder, 2022). Thinking about your attachment styles in particular can be helpful in recognising that you and your partner have a set of expectations about what the other 'should' be like and what a relationship 'ought' to be like. Knowing this helps you stand back and notice your default behaviour. If each of you understands what triggers your tendencies to act a certain way, you have a better chance of stopping the usual cycle of conflict. Couples therapy can help you notice and name the pattern, pause before reacting in the usual way and think about other ways to respond that don't involve criticism, contempt, defensiveness or stonewalling (Gottman, 2007).

Summing it up

Perhaps the most important point is that no one treatment works for every issue or every person. Similarly, as we've seen, there are no NICE guidelines for some of the problems we most frequently face. It's hardly surprising, given the complexity of the human mind.

But given what we do know, let's sum up. First, your preferences matter and choosing a therapy that makes sense to you will make a real difference to the outcome you get. So, tune into your preferences; take time and space to think. Therapy won't work if it doesn't suit you. You need to turn up and stick with it – so don't choose a type of therapy that makes that even harder.

Second, take the available evidence seriously. If you have a specific problem for which there is a clearly recommended treatment, you should consider what NICE says carefully. But look for other sources of advice and guidance too. Websites and charities that specialise in the issues you are dealing with are useful sources of information. As are the websites of the main professional bodies representing counsellors and therapists, and the online therapist directories.

But before you make your choice, there is one final piece of the jigsaw missing. Best practice is made up of three parts: 1) your preferences; 2) the best available evidence, and 3) *the expertise of your therapist* (American Psychological Association, Presidential Task Force on Evidence-Based Practice, 2006). Different therapists get different results. Some therapists are better than others. How to choose the right therapist and get good therapy is the subject of our next chapter.

Ten things to remember

1. No one therapy works for everyone and every problem.
2. Think about your personality and preferences when you choose therapy, and make sure it suits you. You will get much more out of it if you do.
3. Different therapies are good for different things. Short-term therapies can and do help with immediate, pressing problems.

But therapy isn't just about fixing what isn't working. Sometimes you might benefit from more time to explore how you've been impacted by the events of your past.

4. If you want to be challenged, held to account and kept focused, choose a therapy that is strongly goal-focused, sets an agenda and keeps you on topic. If you want a space to talk, feel and think, you'll need a therapy that offers that time and flexibility.
5. Some types of therapy work better than others for particular problems, especially in more complex or severe cases. Bear in mind what the evidence says about different types of therapy and consider that alongside your preferences.
6. Check the research evidence. NICE is the independent body that sifts evidence to determine what works and recommends the best treatments to the NHS. Check its latest guidelines on its website.
7. But be aware that NICE makes recommendations on the basis of cost-effectiveness as well as clinical effectiveness.
8. NICE recommendations are based on large-scale, quantitative trials. It doesn't use qualitative reports, such as patient/user feedback. Be aware of those parameters when you make your choice.
9. There are many instances where NICE makes no recommendations at all – relationship problems, feeling stuck and anger management are just a few of the most common. In this case, use this chapter to inform your choice.
10. For information about other therapies, look to the websites of the main mental health charities and the professional bodies representing counsellors and psychotherapists. You'll also find information on the websites of the online counselling directories.

Chapter 5
What makes good therapy?

Good therapy depends on what you want or need. It's a bit like choosing where to go for a meal out. If you're looking for a Friday night takeaway, then the local pizza place might be perfect. You might want somewhere that offers a more sophisticated menu for an important occasion. And, just as there are some basics that all good restaurants have in common, good therapy is the same.

But a good *meal* depends on the ingredients, the recipe *and* the skill of the person cooking it. In the same way, good therapy depends on the techniques used and also the skill of the therapist.

Good therapy and good therapists go together; they are two sides of the same coin. Some studies (Wampold & Brown, 2005) have shown that the most skilled 25% of therapists are twice as effective as those in the least skilled 25%. Choosing the right therapist will determine whether the help you get is really helpful.

Choosing a good therapist

Some therapists really are better than others. Just as some surgeons are better than others and some athletes are faster than others. When it comes to therapists, several studies (Kraus et al., 2016) confirm large differences between the best and worst, even when they are all delivering the same highly structured treatment (Owen et al., 2019). In other words, the recipe and the ingredients were the same in those studies; the only difference was the skill of the cook.

In fact, the difference is even more stark. The worst therapists can actually cause harm. It's not simply that some therapists are ineffective: the clients of the worst therapists actually deteriorated (Moyers & Miller, 2012). In one study (Okiishi et al., 2003) involving 1841 clients, three therapists had an improvement rate eight times greater than the average therapists.

It's bad enough wasting your time and money on someone who doesn't help you or make any difference; it's quite another to pay good money to a therapist who makes you feel worse than you were before you started. That's why it's crucial to choose a therapist who knows what they are doing and is good at their job.

What qualities should you look for in your therapist?

Let's quickly bust a myth before we get into the details of what you should look for. You might assume that the best therapist is the most experienced, the most highly qualified or the most expensive. In fact, Chow and colleagues (2015) found no evidence that age, years of experience or qualification level had any effect on client outcomes. Similarly, characteristics such as gender make no difference either.

In other words, what you pay or where you go isn't a guarantee of quality. What matters more than a wood-panelled office, smart suit or receding hairline are the personal qualities of your therapist. We outline those qualities below.

Fortunately, researchers have been looking at the question of what makes for a good therapist for some time. While there are differences of emphasis and sometimes different terms used, we know from respected sources (Wampold et al., 2017) that effective therapists convey understanding, authenticity and expertise. Below, we draw on the work of two prominent academics (Miller & Moyers, 2021) to offer a longer list of the eight characteristics that research says are to be found in the best therapists. Let's step through them one by one.

1. Empathy – the ability to enter your frame of reference

A good therapist can see things from your point of view. They can see the world through your eyes. That doesn't mean that they feel the same as you, or that they know exactly how you are feeling, or that they have been through the same experience. 'Accurate empathy', as the term is sometimes labelled, means they work hard to understand what it is like for you, and they reflect that experience back to you in a way that makes sense. In other words, they 'get' you. They understand what you are experiencing.

Sometimes that means your therapist will help you describe something that is hard to talk about. For example, they might prompt you to say a bit more, or they might help you distinguish between anger and anxiety to get to the root of the problem. They will stay silent long enough to listen to your responses, but they'll also let you know they've heard and understood you.

They may also ask you questions about what you have not said. Sure, your partner behaves in an unreasonable way when you argue, but what do *you* do? Do you slam doors, go off in a sulk or silently seethe? Similarly, if you take all the blame yourself, they will ask about your partner's behaviour: are they really such a saint that everything is entirely your fault? A good therapist enables you to see things you don't immediately notice yourself.

In a medical context, we know that empathy is strongly associated with patient satisfaction (Kortlever et al., 2019). It's no different in therapy. In a meta-analysis of more than 6000 clients (Elliott et al., 2018), empathy had a moderate to strong association with clients getting better outcomes from therapy.

2. Non-judgemental acceptance

Your therapist should be able to listen without judgement or condemnation. They should be respectful and sympathetic. Acceptance is about refraining from judgement and listening without blame or shame, both of which generally cause defensiveness and prevent change.

Acceptance doesn't mean being resigned to something or assuming you can't do anything to change your situation. Quite the opposite. Acceptance means being willing to take an honest look at the issue. It doesn't mean playing it down, pretending it isn't as bad as it is and looking on the bright side. A good therapist will help you look at your problem honestly and then decide what to do. Non-judgemental acceptance doesn't mean your therapist is passive. The best therapists challenge their clients (London Centre for Applied Psychology, 2022), but they do so respectfully and in the context of a trusting relationship.

Part of the reason empathy and acceptance are valued so highly by clients in repeated surveys (Barkham et al., 2021b) is that being listened to is so rare in everyday life. More often than not, the person 'listening' is actually just waiting to speak. They will jump in, make assumptions, offer their opinion or start talking about a similar experience they've had. They may even give you advice you haven't asked for. Or they may try to cheer you up, talk you out of the problem, or encourage you to look on the bright side. Genuine acceptance of how you're feeling or thinking is rare in everyday life. A good therapist leaves you feeling that you are someone worth listening to, that your thoughts, feelings and point of view really do matter.

Interestingly, in the same survey, the positive impact of acceptance increased in step with the proportion of ethnic minority people in the sample, suggesting that an accepting style is even more important for those less accustomed to such treatment.

3. Affirming and validating

This is sometimes also called 'warmth' or 'positive regard'. A good therapist will appreciate and affirm things about you that you may have lost sight of. They will validate and normalise your struggles, without minimising them.

And they will draw your attention to your capabilities and strengths, irrespective of the predominance of your problems. This is not about shallow or empty affirmations that can backfire or sound hollow. A good therapist will highlight your genuine qualities and strengths. They will point out and underline the things you are doing right, despite your difficulties.

For many clients, having attention drawn to the positive things about them can be difficult to accept at first. But in time, being appreciated, perhaps for the first time, can be a profound experience. So too can the experience of being genuinely listened to. A good therapist pays attention to, and cares about, the details of your life. By doing so, they convey that you are someone worth listening to. Some studies (Linehan et al., 2002) have found that simple acts of validation can be as effective as evidence-based interventions, even in helping clients with profound problems such as substance misuse. In the Linehan study, basic acts of validation and evidence-based behavioural interventions were both found to be similarly effective in reducing opiate use after 16 months of treatment, and at a later follow-up.

The same research quoted above also shows that, more generally, many people entering therapy need to feel validated before they can move on to specific problem-solving techniques. More generally, meta-analyses (Farber et al., 2018) – analyses of the amalgamated results of large numbers of studies – reveal a strong link between affirmation and positive regard and good outcomes from therapy.

4. Genuineness

Therapists are not meant to be impartial observers. A good therapist is emotionally engaged and will tell you what they are thinking. They are on your side and involved in your problems. We know from research in medicine (Rollnick et al., 2009) that the patients of doctors with good relationship skills who listen well are more likely to follow their advice and therefore have better health outcomes. The same is true for therapy.

Good therapists will observe professional boundaries, of course, but the most competent will share their own experiences with you when they think it will help. This has been associated with forming a better relationship and getting better outcomes for their clients (Hill et al., 2018). Of course, there will also be times when your therapist needs to listen or chooses to stay quiet. Genuineness can be hard to describe but is often easy to spot. So too is its opposite – phoniness. A good therapist makes sure that nothing they say sounds contrived or rehearsed.

A meta-analysis in 2018 (Kolden et al., 2018) found a moderately strong link between good therapy outcomes and genuineness. Remember, we wouldn't expect every skill to have a strong effect on its own. No one skill is a silver bullet; each should be practised alongside the others in this list.

5. Focus

Effective therapists work with you to find a focus for therapy and develop clear goals and a plan for achieving them (Imel & Wampold, 2008). Together, you are trying to tease out what brought you to therapy and what you hope to get from it. Sometimes that is crystal clear ('I want to stop drinking'); other times, less so ('I've lost my direction since my relationship ended'). If the goal isn't immediately obvious, then the first task of therapy is to clarify that. When goals are agreed, progress is much more likely (Tryon & Winograd, 2011). But if your therapist does not help you focus and set goals, then therapy is much less likely to be useful and can end up feeling aimless.

The benefits of goal-setting on performance are one of the most robust and replicable findings in psychological research (Locke et al., 1981). So, find yourself a therapist who is able to help you define and achieve your goals. Your therapist shouldn't just assume that they know what you want from therapy: they should help you articulate this. One study (Swift & Callahan, 2009b) found that, while therapists thought they knew their clients' goals for therapy, this was accurate in less than a third of cases. It's a pretty significant finding, given that we also know that client–therapist agreement on the focus of therapy predicts better outcomes (Tryon & Winograd, 2011).

6. Promoting hope and optimism

Just as it really matters that *you* believe in the therapy you are getting, it also matters that *your therapist* believes in what they are doing *and* in your ability to change. In other words, the placebo effect – where your symptoms improve even when you're given a sugar pill instead of medication – works both ways. In one study (Miller & Tonigan, 1997), therapists were allocated clients trying to stay sober, and were told that some had high potential for recovery. In reality, their likelihood of recovery was no different from that of the other clients in the study. Nevertheless, at the end of treatment, their therapists rated them as being more motivated, more cooperative and showing better signs of staying sober. And the really interesting thing is that, 12 months later, follow-up data confirmed that those same clients really did have higher rates of abstinence from alcohol, plus they were more likely to be employed.

In one way, this study just confirms the age-old placebo effect. But it specifically confirms that therapists are also subject to the placebo effect and that their expectations can become self-fulfilling prophecies. What it means in practice is that your therapist needs to believe in your ability to change and in the power of therapy to help you do so. It means they know that what they practise has been well researched and that they see their own clients getting better on a regular basis. Inspiring hope is part of your therapist's job.

Of course, there is a balance to be struck. You don't want a therapist who makes false promises or who raises unrealistic expectations. But you should expect them to talk to you in positive, hopeful terms. Just as we value optimism in teachers, coaches, parents and friends, it's a quality we should look for in our therapists too.

7. Solution-focused and strengths-based

Your therapist might choose to highlight your strengths and your resilience, especially as you may be coming to therapy at a time when you've lost belief in yourself. Even when things are tough, it is worth recognising the ways in which you have coped or even just hung in there. Where you have made mistakes, you have recognised that and you are now trying to get help, via therapy. Even if you have tried therapy before, here you are again, not giving up. Even when life is at its most difficult, there are usually things worth being grateful for. There may even be signs of hope on the horizon. Your therapist can help you see things that you've lost sight of.

A good therapist will normalise, but not minimise, your problems. This includes letting you know that you are not alone. For example, we know that, on average, one in four people will experience a mental health problem of some kind each year in England (Mind, 2020), and one in six experience what's called a common mental health problem (like anxiety and depression) in any given week (Mind, 2020). It can help to know that.

You might come to therapy thinking that your brain is 'broken' in some way. A good therapist will explain that, in evolutionary terms, the number one job of the brain is to make sure you stay alive, and while this is often useful, the world isn't anywhere near as dangerous as it was 10,000 years ago. We can't turn our brain off, but we can accept how it operates and carry on with our life anyway. It is quite possible to ask someone out, give a speech or confront a co-worker while feeling nervous and experiencing an increased heart rate and a dry mouth. A good therapist will explain that the brain is constantly scanning the world around you for threats, that signals from the brain show up as physiological symptoms, and that they can be ignored when it's safe to do so.

None of that ought to feel like an attempt to minimise your problems, of course. But a good therapist will help you to take perspective, stand back and see the whole picture: the good and the bad. Your therapist should also help you to understand that you are part of an incredibly resilient species. The truth is, we bounce back after all sorts of misfortunes (Bonanno, cited in Brookman-Byrne, 2022). Research with war veterans, abuse survivors, and even the victims of 9/11 shows that trauma is not the natural response to stress (Bonanno, 2021). Our natural response is actually resilience. Although post-traumatic stress and PTSD may be the better-known terms, nearly 90% of survivors report at least one aspect of post-traumatic *growth* (Tedeschi & Calhoun, 1996), such as a renewed appreciation for life, plus a greater sense of their own strength or sense of new possibilities. This compares with ranges of 10–40% of trauma survivors who develop PTSD (Sareen, 2014).

As a species, we are far more resilient than we assume. Sure, therapy is about understanding what has gone wrong, but it's also about what you want to build on and how to do more of what brings you pleasure and makes life worth living. So, a good therapist should ask you about the things you are already doing that you want to increase and expand on. Your situation won't improve if your therapist focuses only on your negative thoughts and emotions. Your therapist should take your problems seriously, but they should focus on your strengths, skills and resilience too.

Because they believe in your resilience, a good therapist will challenge you. Sometimes they might invite you to take another perspective, or they might check you are describing your feelings fully and accurately. For example, you might say you were frustrated by the way your boss spoke to you at work. Your therapist might check back if in fact you were furious about the way your boss spoke to you in front of other team members or an important client. You might say something is 'obvious' to your therapist and they might say that it's not so obvious to them and ask you to explain. If you are ranting or talking non-stop, they might ask you to pause, breathe, ground yourself and come back to the point or the previously agreed focus.

8. Advice and guidance

Your therapist is not simply a neutral observer of your problems. If you are putting yourself down, overlooking your achievements or catastrophising a situation and making it worse than it really is, then it is their role to highlight that. Clearly no one can make you change, but your therapist can and should point out the impact that these negative ways of thinking and behaving has on your life.

Similarly, while they will not impose their opinion on you, a good therapist will give you their advice when it's helpful to you. Doctors, lawyers and financial advisers who merely listen without offering any advice are failing in their duty. Sometimes that's true in therapy too. A good therapist won't tell you what to do, but they may offer you different ways of thinking about your problem, map out scenarios with you, or provide other points of view for you to consider. They might also suggest things that typically help others in a similar situation. At other times, they may simply know practical things that you don't: for example, debt problems can be dealt with if you talk to your creditors when you first get into difficulty, rather than waiting until they escalate to a crisis. Citizens Advice gives free advice and support on consumer rights, claiming benefits, immigration, housing and more; one of the most effective and inexpensive ways to overcome alcoholism is by attending Alcoholics Anonymous meetings (Project MATCH, 1993). Sharing such things can have a profound impact and withholding such information makes little sense. The decision to take or leave any advice is still yours.

This also means that a good therapist is not always silent, despite the outdated cliché of the brooding analyst sitting behind the couch where the client can't actually see them. A good therapist listens carefully and knows how to give you space and time, but they also know that, if they aren't responsive, they can come across as cold, aloof and lacking in concern. If you are continually met with silence when you disclose difficult things to your therapist, it may start to feel awkward and leave you wondering if what you've said has been understood and accepted. A good therapist won't routinely leave you feeling that way.

They can also use their own language as a model, avoiding phrases like 'always' and 'never'. They might invite you to consider what you'd say to a friend in a similar situation: would you really be as harsh as you are being on yourself? They might help you notice your automatic responses to certain situations and help you count the cost of that behaviour. They might suggest things that have worked for others in similar situations. In other words, your therapist will point things out and give you options, but they'll leave it to you to decide. You could think of them as a 'tour guide': they don't tell you what to do, but they don't just follow you around either.

There is clear evidence (Cooper et al., 2019) that the vast majority of clients want a therapist who guides them. We also know that the majority of people get more out of therapy when they get the kind of help they want. Research (Swift et al., 2018) shows a good association between what clients say they want and how well they do in therapy. That analysis, based on 53 studies and more than 16,000 clients, shows that accommodating preferences is associated with more positive outcomes and fewer drop-outs. For most of us, an active therapist who guides us in the right direction is generally the most useful.

In addition to these eight characteristics of a good therapist identified in the research, we offer a ninth: a good therapist should be grounded in the evidence in their field. They should understand the evidence for the problem you seek help with, or find out more about it if you raise something that they aren't expert in. That is a requirement specified in the ethical frameworks of the main professional bodies for therapy and counselling. Just as you would expect a medical professional to be able to explain why they are recommending a particular course of action and the likely outcomes and any risks, you should expect this from your therapist too.

The psychotherapy literature contains nearly 100 years of research and more than four decades of rigorous, large-scale trials. If your prospective therapist isn't knowledgeable about that, then we recommend you look for someone else. If a therapist is dismissive of the evidence, it means they are making decisions on the basis of their personal preferences or how they've always done things. You wouldn't accept a nurse or doctor being uninformed about the latest evidence regarding a physical health problem. You shouldn't accept it in relation to your mental health either. Checking out their knowledge and familiarity with the basic evidence base for therapy is one of the quickest ways you can establish whether you are seeing someone who is serious about their work and serious about helping you.

Your preferences still matter

Of course, each of those eight qualities needs to be kept in balance and to be practised alongside the others. Too much optimism or focus on solutions with too little empathy will likely leave you feeling your experience hasn't been validated or understood. Too much acceptance of the difficulty you are in and not enough focus on your strengths or guidance about options for moving forward may leave you feeling hopeless. Practised in the right measure and blended together, the qualities above become more than the sum of their parts.

Nevertheless, you may know from the outset that some qualities are more important to you than others. For example, you might know that you need the emphasis to be on validation and affirmation. Conversely, you may know that a focus on your strengths and resilience is the best way to overcome the challenge you face. If so, take that seriously. As we saw in the previous chapter, your preferences matter. The qualities above are borne out by research and are time-honoured interpersonal qualities, but they still need to be tailored to you.

While studies show that some therapists are better than others, you still need to find a therapist who fits with what *you* need. Even the best therapists don't work equally well with everyone in their caseload. In other words, what works for one client won't necessarily work for you. 'Fit', 'chemistry' and 'matching' are still important. The best therapists are able to flex their style, but they can't be all things to all people or serve everyone equally well.

While some therapists may be better than others on average, *you* are not average, and the trick is to find the best therapist for you. Research (Spencer et al., 2019) indicates that therapist–client compatibility plays a significant role in the outcome of therapy. So, keep in mind the particular qualities that are important to you when you are choosing your therapist.

Next, we walk through the practical steps involved in selecting a therapist and we highlight what to look out for to ensure the best fit.

Where to look and what for

Check out the online directories that list therapists who belong to a recognised professional body. Unless you have a personal recommendation, this is a good place to start your search. A Google search for 'therapy-therapist/counselling-counsellor near me' will bring up the current most well-used directory sites. Or you could use the 'Find a therapist' search function on the two main UK online directories, *www.welldoing.org* and *www.counselling-directory.org.uk*, and the websites of the main PSA-accredited professional bodies: the UK Council for Psychotherapy (*www.psychotherapy.org.uk*), the British Association for Psychotherapy and Counselling BACP) (*www.bacp.co.uk*), the British Psychological Society (BPS) (*www.bps.org.uk*), and the National Counselling & Psychotherapy Society (NCS) (*https://nationalcounsellingsociety.org*).

These directory listings include a basic description of your potential therapist, what kind of therapy they provide and their areas of experience/expertise. You can usually search by type of therapy you would prefer. The listing should also tell you a bit about their background, qualifications, the type of therapy they provide, what they specialise in and where they are based. Some therapists work online *and* in-person. Others do one or the other. Maddeningly for many potential clients, therapists often don't include information on their fees and you may need to phone or email to find this out. Nor do they always state if their premises are accessible to disabled people and in what ways (ground floor, ramp, lift, accessible toilet etc.).

Most therapists also have their own website (although a surprising number don't). Taking a look at the website will give you more of a 'feel' for how they work and who they are and it may include more detailed information, such as cancellation policies and how they record, store and use your data.

As well as looking at the factual information on the directory listing and the website, ask yourself if you can get a sense of what the therapist is like. What 'tone' are they giving off? Do they seem open, professional, reassuring, warm? Is the information clear, organised and helpful? It's generally considered unethical for therapists to post client testimonials and reviews on their social media pages and websites, so don't be put off if you can't find many reviews for your preferred choice. Try to think about the qualities that are most important to you and ask yourself if this is the kind of person you can imagine talking and opening up to. If not, keep looking: there are tens of thousands of therapists in private practice in the UK. Don't just pick one; identify a handful and then it's time to reach out to them directly.

With some therapists, you can book and pay for a session up-front online, assuming you're satisfied that they offer what you need. But you might want to talk to them first. Sometimes an email exchange will be enough, but most therapists offer a free 10–15-minute consultation, usually on the phone or online. This is your opportunity to ask about anything that isn't clear or that you'd like them to expand on. They will probably ask you to briefly share your problem. Remember, this isn't a therapy session and you won't have time to tell them everything about yourself or your problem. Outline the most important points as best you can. Try to be as honest and open as you can. It's quite normal to be nervous. A good therapist will let you know whether or not they are experienced in dealing with your issue and whether they think they can help.

Apart from exploring the practicalities, such as availability and cost, this initial meeting is also your opportunity to assess whether you think they are the right person for you. What is it like to talk to this person? Are they warm, thoughtful, reassuring, understanding and professional? Did they put you at your ease? Research suggests (Ardito & Rabellino, 2011) that the relationship between the therapist and the client is among the most important factors influencing the outcomes of therapy, so take your first impressions seriously. Talk to a few different therapists before making your final decision. Assuming they are all properly trained and qualified, research suggests that it's best to base the decision on how the interaction 'feels', because there is such strong evidence that an effective working relationship with your therapist is so central to effective therapy (American Psychological Association, 2019).

Initial session

If an initial call has gone well and you've decided to meet with one of your short-listed therapists, the best and really only way to tell if they are a good fit is to go ahead and book a first session. Some therapists offer this session for free (although most don't – few professionals will give away an hour of their time for free, after all). Obviously, you are checking the basics: Are they on time? Is the room clean, comfortable, quiet and private? Or, if the session was online, did the technology work and could you see and hear them clearly? But beyond the basics, you are also checking for the qualities described in this chapter: Were they attentive? Did they seem genuine and empathetic? Did you feel validated? Did they seem to understand your problem and guide the session somewhere helpful?

Perhaps most importantly, have you started to build a rapport with them that makes you think you'd want to see them again? In short, do you trust them to help you? While you need to feel at ease with a therapist, the 'nicest' or warmest therapist may not be the most effective in the long run. If you're like the majority of people, you also want someone who will challenge you, guide you and keep you focused. Think back to your favourite teacher. They had time for you and were on your side, but they probably didn't let you sell yourself short. They might have even 'pushed' you on occasions or had a reputation for being 'strict'. Make sure your therapist leaves you feeling that they know what they are doing and are likely to be good at their job. You are not looking to employ a 'well-paid friend'.

Sometimes the first session will be enough to convince you that you've found the right person. Other times, you might need another couple of sessions to be sure. In some instances, the first session won't feel quite right, and you may come out knowing that you need to continue the search. In many ways, that was the point, so don't be afraid to cut your losses. Research confirms (Erekson et al., 2020) that differences in therapists' effectiveness are often evident in the first session and that this predicts their clients' outcomes. It's often a better use of money and time to quit after one session if the connection doesn't feel right.

But similarly, if the first session goes well and you get a good feel from your new therapist, don't be afraid to commit. Go with your gut. If the interaction feels good, go for it. The sooner you start therapy, the sooner you will start to see the benefits. Beginning therapy requires you to take a calculated risk, as does pretty much everything else worthwhile in life.

In other words, don't waste time looking for the 'perfect' therapist. Your therapist doesn't need to be perfect. The task is to start working on changes that are important to you, with someone helpful beside you, not to find the best therapist in town. So, give your 'good-enough' therapist a chance. They can't read your mind, so ask your questions, share any misgivings and let them know your preferences. See how they respond. Don't sabotage the opportunity to get 'good-enough' help by expecting them to meet impossibly high standards. Does it really matter if their room is a little messy, parking is a bit difficult, or their dress sense is a little 'off'? If the relational (and technological) connection is good enough, get started.

The principles of good therapy

Once you've found a good-enough therapist, how do you know if you're getting good therapy? One of the best and simplest ways to think about what comprises good therapy is to consider the principles of change that are shared across all the main forms of therapy (Pachankis & Goldfried, 2007). We list below what many people consider to be the five principles that lead to change in psychotherapy:

1. Good therapy depends on you and your therapist believing that it will help

One of the key elements of successful therapy is that you believe it will change something about your life for the better. Research finds this to be true time and time again (Bartholomew et al., 2021), most obviously in medicine, where the placebo effect shows how powerful your thoughts and expectations are. Having confidence that something will help you usually means that it does.

As we've discussed above, in therapy you gain that confidence by working with a therapist who inspires your trust and gives you a realistic sense that they can help you because they have helped others in a similar situation. Your therapist's job is to convey that optimism to you. Good therapy feels hopeful.

2. Good therapy requires a good working relationship with your therapist

If you don't trust or respect your therapist, then it's unlikely you'll get much out of therapy. Similarly, if you feel they don't 'get you', or if they speak down to you or confuse you, that will not lead to an effective working partnership.

The good news is you can usually tell this very early on. If you detect problems in the first few sessions, don't ignore them or hope for the best. Whatever the issue is, raise it with your therapist, give them a chance to respond, but if they don't, it's time to look elsewhere. It's not going to be possible to be honest about the most difficult aspects of your life with someone you don't trust or respect or feel comfortable with.

3. Good therapy improves your awareness of what's going on in your life

That includes the way your mind tends to work and how you tend to be in your relationships, whether with bosses, partners, friends, children or parents. Your therapist's job is to help you see when you overreact or when you are inflexible or impulsive or you assume you know exactly what others are thinking. Your therapist can help you stand back and spot things you can't see for yourself.

It can be uncomfortable to have your views challenged or your 'flaws' pointed out. At times, your therapist might make observations or ask questions that feel challenging. Therapy is not always fun. It's meant to help you change something about your life. And the first step to that is noticing when you do things on autopilot that are not in your best interests. Once that's in place, you can often make rapid changes (Gingerich & Peterson, 2013).

4. Therapy is an opportunity to do things differently

Improved awareness of how you think and act is step one, but it's not enough. In time, it will also mean doing things differently. That might be speaking up at work or asking the guy at the gym to go for coffee. Either way, it's making a deliberate choice to act differently, in the hope of a better outcome. If you want change, you will have to take a risk and behave differently.

Good therapy makes sure those changes are at a speed and intensity you can tolerate. Like a good fitness programme, therapy should feel challenging but not overwhelming. Working with a good therapist is a lot like working with a personal trainer. In both cases, they assess what you are ready for and won't suggest more than they think you can handle. But they are also in your corner, encouraging you to work hard and sometimes do uncomfortable things. In the end, whether you do them or not is up to you. And, as with physical exercise, outcomes in therapy are largely determined by the effort you put in.

5. Tie it all together into a virtuous circle

Therapy helps you link increased awareness of the things you want to change with a new experience of doing them differently. This means recognising something that you are avoiding or noticing a pattern that you have been repeating on autopilot, and then doing something differently to break that cycle. Often this produces a different and better outcome, which results in you thinking that it was a risk worth taking.

Even when the risks don't pay off – your boss rejects your proposal or the guy you ask out for a coffee says no – you realise it's not the end of the world. You might well still feel proud you took the risk, and you might be more inclined to do so again. Good therapy helps you realise that you really do miss 100% of the shots you don't take.

While the stereotype of therapy is that it focuses on your childhood and the pain of your past, good therapy is every bit as much focused on the future and getting on with living. What do you want to do more of and build on? How did you get through previous tough times? Can you identify the smallest change that you can quickly put into practice to improve your life? When you've done so, can you recognise those improvements, give yourself credit, and build on them? Over and over?

Summing it up

Good therapy can't be separated from the therapist who delivers it. Different therapists get very different results. Not only are some better than others, but the worst therapists can make you feel worse. And this has nothing to do with age, experience or training; it's about their interpersonal qualities.

Research suggests you should be looking for a therapist who is empathic, non-judgemental, validating, genuine, focused on your goals and willing to challenge you to reach them; one who believes in your resilience, builds on your strengths and is committed to guiding you towards solutions that work for you. A good therapist blends and balances those characteristics.

Your preferences matter too. If you know that some qualities are more important to you than others, take that seriously when choosing your therapist.

Clearly, you also need someone properly trained and registered with a recognised professional body or statutory register. Online directories are the most convenient way of finding them and are a useful first port of call.

But don't let the search for the perfect therapist be the enemy of finding one who is good enough. The only way to really tell if a therapist is right for you is to go ahead with the first session. Did you feel understood? Did they seem genuine? Have you started to build a rapport? Were there any red flags? If so, don't be afraid to cut your losses and move on.

The aim is not to find the perfect therapist. The aim is to find someone who can help you make changes that enable you to live a better life.

At its best, therapy can change your life. So, it's important that you get the best therapy you can. In the end, however, its effectiveness depends on the amount of effort you put in. Your therapist can't and won't fix you on their own – we'll look at your own readiness and motivation in more detail in Chapter 9.

At the other end of the spectrum, the worst therapists can cause you harm. They can reduce your trust in other people; they can make you leave therapy despite not getting the benefits; they can make you feel you are to blame for your own problems. And there are therapists who are simply just not that good at their job. You'll end therapy with them feeling no better, having wasted your time and money. So in the next chapter, we discover what bad therapy looks like, why there is so much of it and how you can avoid it.

Ten things to remember

1. Good therapy can't be separated from the therapist who delivers it. Different therapists get different results and the

worst therapists can actually leave you feeling worse than when you started.

2. The best therapists are empathic, non-judgemental, affirming, genuine, focused on your goals, hopeful, solution-focused and willing to act as a guide.
3. The differences between the best and worst therapists have nothing to do with age, experience, gender or the type of therapy they practise.
4. Even though some therapists are better than others, what works for one client won't work for everyone. You need to choose the right therapist for *you*.
5. Research shows that the relationship between therapist and client is one of the most important factors influencing the outcomes of therapy.
6. When making your choice, use online directories that list registered therapists' professional qualifications and accreditation, and check out therapists' own websites to find out what they offer and to get a 'feel' for who they are.
7. Most therapists offer a free initial telephone/online consultation. Make use of it to ask any questions you may have.
8. After the first session, take time to review how you experienced it. Did you feel understood and at ease? If not, don't be afraid to cut your losses, move on and find another therapist.
9. But your therapist doesn't need to be perfect. Good enough is good enough. Raise any questions, misgivings and preferences with them and see how they respond.
10. Remember your role too. More than any other single factor, the effort and commitment you put into therapy make the biggest difference to whether it works or not.

Chapter 6
What does bad therapy look like?

It's as important to be able to spot bad therapy as it is to be able to spot good therapy. Bad therapy will cost you time and money and energy. If you're lucky, it might not have helped but it won't have caused harm either. You'll end therapy feeling no better, but you will have wasted your time and money.

If you're unlucky, bad therapy can make things worse.

The therapy industry – what you need to know

When you go to a doctor, the chances are that they'll talk you through a limited number of very similar options for your treatment. Should you take ibuprofen, paracetamol or codeine for your pain? Do you have the operation that will fix your problem, given the risks involved, or do you wait a few months and see how the pills help?

You wouldn't expect your doctor to say, 'There are 100 different ways to treat your diabetes.' You wouldn't expect your personal trainer to say, 'There are 100 different ways of getting stronger and losing weight.'

Therapy shouldn't be any different. But unfortunately it is. Yes, most of the time you'll find yourself sitting in a room (or in front of a screen) with a person who listens to you, validates your feelings, shows compassion and offers advice, guidance and support. But the therapy itself might be any one of hundreds of different interventions.

A big reason for this is that the therapy industry is a mess. There are more than 500 different types of therapy (Lilienfeld & Arkowitz,

2012). Literally anyone can set up a business and call themselves a psychotherapist, counsellor or executive/life coach. They don't need to have done a single minute of relevant training. And there are myriad trainings, at all levels, from Certificate through to Master's and on to PhD. So, we suggest you look for a therapist who at the very least has been through training that has been accredited by one of the main professional bodies, such as the UK Council for Psychotherapy (UKCP), the National Counselling & Psychotherapy Society (NCS) or the British Association for Counselling and Psychotherapy (BACP).

Compare that approach with going to see a medical doctor. You can expect all GPs to have pretty much the same training, regardless of where they trained. Your doctor can't use their work as an opportunity to test out their wacky ideas of what's going to help you. They have to implement evidence-based treatments or they will get struck off the General Medical Council's register. The brain is the most complex organ in the human body. We're still in the very early days of understanding how it works. But, rather than that understanding leading to caution, we have an industry that allows anyone to meddle with your mind, using techniques that could be based simply on their own pet theory.

Some therapies are short-lived fads, some are endorsed by celebrities but have little evidence to support them, some are recommended by NICE for use in the NHS. And you need a way to help you sift through them and find one that will work for you and your problems.

Market forces in any industry incentivise the bold and the new. Tried and tested evidence-based techniques don't seem as exciting. They don't sell as many books or conference tickets. You want to feel like you're getting the newest treatments. But in the psychotherapy world, the reality is that they may well be entirely untested and sold to you on the basis of first-person testimony alone.

Avoiding a bad therapist

Most therapists are prone to believing they're better than they are. That just makes them human. Cognitive biases like unrealistic optimism lead more than 90% of us to think we're better than average drivers (Svenson, 1981). But that's impossible: only 50% by definition can be above average at anything. Only 50% of therapists are above average. While you're more likely to find a good therapist if you search for those who are registered with a professional body that is accredited by the Professional Standards Authority (PSA), some will still be unreliable and poor practitioners. We suggest you walk away from therapy with anyone who:

- **gets fundamental practicalities wrong** – they forget your sessions. Or they frequently start sessions late or end them early. They routinely bill you incorrectly and/or late. They regularly cancel your sessions at short notice. If you're working with them online, they have internet difficulties, or you can't hear them or see them well. Your mental health is too important to trust it to someone who can't even get the basics right. Even if the therapist seems kind and supportive, if they can't also be reliable and predictable, look elsewhere.
- **allows therapy to go on too long** – most therapists want to help you. But they also have a financial incentive to keep you coming to see them. Don't let your therapist become a well-paid friend. Make sure you're only in therapy for as long as you feel you need to be. If you feel your therapist is constantly straying off topic, ask them to come back to your goals, and insist you have regular reviews to see how you are progressing towards achieving them. Of course, therapy doesn't always have to be goal oriented. There may well be times in your life when you just want someone to talk to, once a week or fortnight, to help you process how you think and feel and offer advice and support. But if that's the case, make sure it's on your terms.
- **is too passive** – a lot of what you'll gain from therapy is from having someone listen to you, offer compassionate understanding and sympathy and allow you space to process how you feel. But people often benefit from challenge and focus too. Sometimes you may need someone to encourage you out of your comfort zone and keep you moving towards your goals, to help you see what you're capable of, even when you're struggling to see that yourself. If therapy feels a little too easy or cosy, it's possible that your therapist isn't working you hard enough or isn't working hard enough on your behalf.

- **is unfocused** – the best therapists will, from the first session, help you get to the heart of what's contributing to your distress and will help you understand what you can do to start feeling better. That won't necessarily be immediate, and there might be some false starts and wrong turns along the way. But you should feel that you're working with your therapist towards that understanding. If you're left feeling you've waffled through 50 minutes without any sense of direction or structure and without much help along the way, it may be time to consider a different therapist.
- **makes you feel uncomfortable and awkward** – let's be honest, therapy can be awkward. You're meeting a stranger, often in their house, to talk about your most intimate and embarrassing problems. They often see you at your worst. That's uncomfortable. You don't want your therapist's manner and behaviour to add to that discomfort. That's not to dismiss individuality: the best therapists bring their personalities, quirks and even eccentricities to their work with you. But if your therapist can't put you at ease or makes you feel consistently awkward, then you're best off looking elsewhere.
- **uses too much jargon** – too many therapists use language that is strange and confusing to the ordinary punter. If they can't explain clearly what they are doing and why it will be helpful, then possibly they don't really know what they're doing or don't understand it themselves. You have a right to expect a therapist to be able to explain things in simple, everyday language and to check back with you to make sure you've understood.
- **leaves you feeling worse after sessions** – you'll often hear therapists say, 'It'll feel worse before it feels better.' What they mean when they say that is something like, 'You've been avoiding this for ages, so confronting it is going to be painful and difficult, but I'm here to help guide you through it at the right speed and in the right way.' However, bad therapists dive right in and hold to the view that if you're feeling something big, crying a lot and breaking down, then something therapeutic is happening. This is pretty much the opposite of best contemporary thinking, which stresses the need for a

staged approach. You shouldn't leave every session feeling like you're in a vulnerable place without any strategies to help you cope with your life after the session. Ideally, your therapist will spend the last few minutes of a session helping you to get back to your normal self.

- **doesn't seem to care about you** – a small minority of therapists churn out CBT worksheets like robots, insist on giving you homework when you don't want it, or get up and draw on a whiteboard, which reminds you of being back at school. Others sit silent, unresponsive and expressionless as you pour your heart out. You need a therapist who you *know* cares about you; you can feel it, even when they don't say it.
- **is too much of a cheerleader** – the opposite of the uncaring therapist is the therapist who tells you only what they think you want to hear: positive affirmations and validations of all your feelings. Your therapist isn't meant to be your friend or parent. They're there to help you, and that sometimes involves telling you what is difficult to hear, in compassionate and constructive ways.
- **focuses on the past without helping you in your present** – your past is crucial to how you feel now. Your early relationships helped shape who you are, how you react in stressful situations and how you act in relationships. Your therapist will help you understand that. But the least effective therapists stay in the past or stay there too long. They don't help you to consider how you can change those learned patterns of behaving and they may keep taking you back again and again to those early relationships. Make sure you're working with a therapist who helps you to get out of the hole as well as to understand how you got into it in the first place.
- **dismisses your preferences** – some therapists think they've got all the answers. They think their approach will work for you, regardless of what you're struggling with. They don't care that you don't want to do homework between sessions. They don't care whether you want more challenge. They are the person with the training and you're the client. Find a therapist who knows that acknowledging your preferences is a crucial

element to helping you – and knows that there is research evidence to prove this.

- **never says 'sorry', 'I don't know', or 'I'll have to think about that and come back to you'** – bad therapists lack humility. They think they know what's best for you. So, in their minds, they can't get anything wrong. If the treatment doesn't help you, then they'll dismiss you as a 'difficult' client who isn't ready for therapy. If you suggest they made a mistake, they will come back at you and make it seem like your fault. Find yourself a therapist who knows they screw up sometimes and is prepared to admit it and learn from it.
- **never answers your questions with a straight answer** – some therapists will make you feel silly for asking simple questions. They will refuse to offer simple advice when you ask, and instead switch the focus to your reasons for asking. Sometimes, your therapist will be right to not give you advice and will challenge you to come to your own decisions, but if your therapist never gives a straight answer to a straight question, you should probably go elsewhere.
- **doesn't do their homework** – some therapists expect their clients to teach them about things they should be finding out for themselves, like cultural issues that are particular to you, or background information around a problem you have brought or an illness you are coping with, or ways to meet your access or communication needs. You are paying them to give you therapy, not to learn from your experience at your expense.

Some interventions make things worse

As well as knowing how to avoid a bad therapist, you need to know which types of therapy to avoid. Some well-intentioned and intuitive therapeutic interventions can make your mental health worse. They may sound like they should work, but they can do damage.

In general, talking about our struggles makes us feel better. As the Royal College of Psychiatrists puts it (2021b), 'Research has shown that talking about the event and your feelings can help you to be more resilient. Avoiding memories and feelings has been shown to make people feel worse.' And mostly, that is true – but not always. In the 1980s and 1990s, a treatment for PTSD called 'psychological debriefing' was developed on the principle that getting people talking as soon as possible about their trauma (for example, following a serious road traffic accident) prevents the onset of longer-term PTSD. However, when it was finally subjected to rigorous research, psychological debriefing was found to have no beneficial effects and potentially to make things worse (Mayou et al., 2000). What was more likely to be of *immediate* help to victims was to be around people who made them feel safe: family and friends. It seems that talking about trauma is most likely to be therapeutic only once our bodies and minds have regained to some degree a sense of safety. And even then, it can quite often turn out not to be necessary.

The 'recovered memory' scandals of the late 20th century caused real harm to thousands of lives. This notion was based on an incorrect understanding about how our brains process and recall memories. A number of therapists argued that their clients' mental health struggles, including depression and eating disorders, were a result of repressed memories of childhood sexual abuse. This resulted in a rash of accusations against parents and other adults about sexual and ritual, satanic abuse. The 'repressed' or 'recovered' memories were believed, despite a lack of supporting evidence. There is now general agreement about the existence of false memories of sexual abuse and that great harm resulted from these beliefs, however genuinely they were held (Brewin & Andrews, 2017).

The Scared Straight treatment programme and 'boot camps' in the United States are another example of an intervention based on an idea that intuitively *seems* right but in practice causes immense damage. The Scared Straight programme tried to reduce crime by exposing young people deemed at risk of criminality to the reality of prison life. Follow-up studies suggested, however, that the young people put through the programme were subsequently more likely to end up in prison (New Zealand Government, 2016).

The likelihood is that some current high-profile, trending treatments will be found to be the same when robust research is done. Many simply won't work: they won't cause harm, but they won't do any good either. What they will do is waste time, effort and resources that could be applied to therapy treatments for which there is robust evidence that they do work. Our advice is to stick to tried and trusted routes down the ski slope, because going off piste can be dangerous.

Each generation has its equivalent of the well-resourced, heavily publicised interventions described above. Novel types of therapy promise incredible results and sometimes even seem to demonstrate them in early studies, often undertaken and published by the originators of the treatments themselves, with very small numbers of participants and no comparators. But more often than not, those treatments end up fizzling out in the following decade because subsequent large-scale research finds them to be neutral, harmful or simply reflecting aspects of existing evidence-based therapy. As was said of one such popular therapy (Arkowitz & Lilienfeld, 2012), 'What is effective in the treatment is not new, and what is new is not effective.'

Types of therapy to avoid

So how do you navigate this confusing mess and avoid bad therapy? One obvious way is to ask questions of your prospective therapist in your initial phone call, and then in more detail during your initial session. You can ask that they suggest articles that summarise the evidence for the approach they use. Do they get defensive when you ask questions about the evidence? Do they simply talk about the good results they personally have achieved with their clients? Ask them if they have experience of working with others with your particular issues. Good therapists know their limits and will be humble enough to refer you elsewhere if they don't have the necessary experience and knowledge to meet your needs.

In terms of sorting through the 500 options for particular approaches, we recommend that you ignore the ones that have a very weak or non-existent research base. Of course, most therapies will have proponents who claim they are 'evidence-based' or 'backed by science.' You find that in many unregulated industries. There are practitioners out there who want to take your money, even when they know they're peddling pseudoscience. You'll also find many more therapists who wholeheartedly believe their way of working is the best way to help you, even if you might get them to acknowledge there is no research evidence to support that claim. Many therapists are content to rely on the anecdotal evidence of their success with their clients as sufficient proof that their way of working is the best for you. You should not be happy to go with that. They might be right: the chances are, they're not.

The boldest and most outlandish claims should provoke your scepticism. These are often the new, exciting treatments that come with brash statements about speedy results. For example, a therapy technique called 'brainspotting' aims to treat trauma by asking you to point your eyes in directions apparently associated with certain memories. The therapist might hold a pencil or a pointer in front of your eyes in various locations to identify a spot in your vision where you feel most 'activated'. They'll then ask you to continue staring at that spot and gently encourage you to recall your traumatic experience.

Despite its growing number of advocates, there is no scientific consensus around the idea that eye movements are linked with specific memories. More importantly, there are no peer-reviewed studies of this intervention where it has been tested against other treatments such as trauma-focused CBT and a control group. If there is neither an understanding of why it works nor a robust research base to support a certain treatment, there's a strong likelihood you'd be wasting your time and money.

Another therapy you've probably heard of, based on similar ideas to brainspotting, is eye movement desensitization and reprocessing therapy (EMDR). It has spawned a whole industry of specialist training and professional development programmes, is offered by thousands of therapists as part of their 'toolkit', and is frequently name-checked by celebrities, including one member of our Royal Family, as having transformed their life. It is particularly lauded for its use in treating post-traumatic stress disorder, and NICE recommends that it should be considered for children and young people and adults if exposure therapy hasn't helped and if the adult expresses a preference for it (which stops short of a full-on endorsement) (NICE, 2018).

EMDR invites you to focus on traumatic memories while simultaneously looking from side to side, either following your therapist's finger or a swinging object, or just looking left and right repeatedly. A similar approach is tapping, where you tap your left and right leg while focusing on traumatic memories. However, the academic consensus (Davidson & Parker, 2001) is that the eye movements in EMDR are unnecessary, and that the effect it achieves is simply the result of recalling the traumatising event, as you would in exposure therapy. In CBT-based exposure, you are invited to gradually confront what you fear with the aim of discovering for yourself that, however unpleasant it is, it is not harmful and you are capable of tolerating the temporary distress it causes. Head-to-head clinical trials consistently show exposure-based CBT to be more effective than EMDR (Salkovskis, 2001). So, let's be clear: EMDR works better than doing nothing, especially for treating trauma, and is better than just supportive listening. But, as some experts consider (Layard & Clark, 2015a), it is probably because EMDR is a form of CBT by another name.

Research you can trust

You can't be expected to sort through the research base for every type of therapy. The vast majority of therapists won't have done that, although all therapists should have a good understanding of the elements that make for good therapy outcomes. Indeed, those who are registered with a PSA-accredited body are required to keep up to date with the evidence in their field, and to evidence this annually. So don't feel shy about asking them to demonstrate that understanding.

Thankfully, there are independent, well-respected organisations out there who have done that job for you. The best are the Cochrane Foundation and NICE (we discussed NICE and its role within the UK public health system in Chapter 4). The Cochrane Foundation is an independent research body that specialises in what they call 'systematic reviews', which review the data and evidence available on a specific topic. The reviews are lodged online in the Cochrane Library.

Of course, you're unlikely to have the time or inclination to search through detailed, often dense guidance, and a lot of the original research will be behind scientific journals' paywalls. But some knowledge of the headlines from the research summaries will help you ascertain if your therapist is familiar with the most up-to-date evidence and guidance.

Summing it up

Good therapy and bad therapy are two sides of the same coin. Good therapists are authentic and make you feel understood and accepted. They shape the work around your preferences and know from current research what is likely to help you with your specific problem. They treat you as resilient and challenge you accordingly, when it's appropriate. They're solution-focused and have a good idea of when the therapy should end.

Bad therapists think the way they work is the best, if not the only way to treat everything. They're dogmatic in how they do things, follow the manual slavishly and are likely to leave you feeling misunderstood and unheard. They are too passive and let you get away with too many excuses, or they apply too much aggressive 'tough love' in the way they challenge you when you're not ready. They let therapy go on forever, even though that's not what you signed up for, and they don't check in with how you feel it's progressing.

So now you know how to spot and avoid bad therapy. But there are alternatives to talking one-to-one with a live therapist in the same room. We are now in the 21st century; Covid-19 has transformed the therapy world by forcing therapists to work online and make more use of digital technology. There's also the growing use of artificial intelligence to power online therapies, and widespread use of apps, especially in the wellbeing industry, offering instant advice day or night, even if it's not from a human.

So, this is what we are going to explore in the next chapter.

Ten things to remember

1. The research is there; we know what good therapy looks like; there are plenty of good therapists out there. You don't need to settle for a bad therapist.
2. Anyone can call themselves a therapist or a counsellor, without having any training or qualifications. And between them they offer 500 different types of therapy, for which in many cases there is no evidence to show they work.

3. To avoid working with someone who is not qualified to help you, choose a therapist who is registered with the UKCP, BACP or NCS. Check their qualifications on the therapist directories – if the therapist doesn't list them, then they likely don't have them.
4. If a therapist is frequently late for appointments or keeps changing the time, doesn't care about your preferences or leaves you feeling worse after every session, look elsewhere.
5. Bad therapists lack humility. They overestimate their ability to help. They underestimate the importance of your experience and checking in with you. They seem robotic. They don't make you feel cared about. Avoid them.
6. If it sounds too good to be true, it probably is. Some therapies promise immediate support for deep-rooted problems. Some therapies offer weird explanations for their mechanisms of action and use outlandish techniques. Stay hopeful that your chosen therapy can help, but retain a healthy scepticism about inflated promises.
7. Don't rely on celebrity anecdotes or endorsements. One anecdote is just one person's experience. It's not a scientifically robust study.
8. A small minority of psychological treatments and interventions actually make things worse. Focus on the treatments that are supported by robust evidence.
9. Ask your therapist in your initial contact or early sessions to describe what they think might be contributing to your distress and how their proposed method is likely to help. Notice any defensiveness on their part. Notice if they rely on anecdotal evidence rather than large-scale studies.
10. The best sources of summaries of the scientific evidence are NICE, via their clinical guidelines, and the Cochrane Foundation's systematic reviews. Search their websites for the relevant evidence summaries and have a conversation with your therapist about the findings. All good therapists should be familiar with the latest research in their field. Be wary if they are not.

Chapter 7
Can technology improve therapy?

Getting therapy in the 21st century is, in general, not that different to how it was throughout the 20th century. You go to a therapist's office, sit in a chair or lie on a couch and get help by talking to a live person who is in the same room. Up until a few years ago, there was no reliable, accessible technology, other than the telephone, to allow you to stay in touch with your therapist when you couldn't make it to their office (or if you simply preferred to be at home).

In some ways, that consistency of approach speaks to the success of therapy. If it ain't broke, don't fix it. As we've seen, there is now a significant body of evidence to show that therapy, practised well, is very helpful for the majority of people. Until recently, few people questioned the fundamentals of therapy. Then came the brutal disruption to our usual lives caused by the Covid-19 pandemic, and the almost overnight embracing of information technology and the internet by the talking therapies professions.

And as a result, therapy is changing fast. From outright hostility at worst and grudging welcome at best, therapists started using online video platforms to work with their clients. Moreover, they have also started using text-only media, such as text, email and instant messaging (Worley-James, 2022). This is generally good news; we have in our homes and in our pockets a device that not only contains the entirety of human knowledge but allows us to connect to other humans at a moment's notice. It would be stupid to ignore the potential benefits of these developments, despite the widespread, often overblown (Vuorre et al., 2021) fears that the internet and social media are destroying our mental health. Other health care industries are embracing these opportunities. Therapy should be no different.

In this chapter, we'll look at the ways therapy is changing rapidly to make good use of these technologies. Most importantly, we'll show you what to trust and what to avoid in this new world. Does having therapy online make any difference to whether it'll help you? How useful is it to experience simulations of difficult situations in your life and practise new skills in a virtual world peopled by avatars? Do chatbots that use artificial intelligence to generate their dialogue offer the same benefits as a living, breathing human being?

Online video/teletherapy

Very few private therapists worked online via video calls before the Covid-19 pandemic. Most preferred to offer sessions from their office or therapy room, which was not infrequently in their own home. This may have been for convenience, but there was also a deep-seated belief that there was something special about the physical presence of two bodies in the same room. Some therapists speak of the 'holding' nature of the therapist's 'presence', and how two bodies being together in the same room, breathing the same air, can be in some way calming for the client and enable them to explore their thoughts and feelings more deeply (Totton, 2015).

To some extent, this makes sense. It can be calming to be near our loved ones, and in the same room when speaking with them. Talking to your family and friends on a video call doesn't replicate the experience of sitting around a table, sharing food and conversation with them. But there is nothing inherently magical about being in the same room as your therapist during therapy. They aren't a good friend or a family member; hugs and physical contact are not a vital element of the therapeutic relationship. Unless you've specifically chosen a therapy based on body contact and movement, you're in therapy to talk, reflect, stand back, broaden your perspective and work hard to improve your life.

And it turns out you can do that online as effectively as you can in person.

The proof is in the research. A meta-analysis (Batastini et al., 2020) of 57 studies, which together totalled more than 4,300 clients, compared in-person therapy with video sessions and found no difference in whether the therapy was helpful or not. A separate review (Luo et al., 2020) of 17 studies, focusing on CBT specifically, found that online therapy for depression may even be more effective than face-to-face sessions. Other research (Irvine et al., 2020) has found little difference in terms of the strength of the therapeutic relationship, the depth of client disclosures or the therapist's levels of empathy or attentiveness when sessions were carried out on the phone. Nevertheless, clients and therapists in the same study did express reservations about the delivery of psychological therapy by telephone. These concerns centred around the quality of the therapeutic relationship and the ability to exercise professional judgement in the absence of visual cues, but no evidence for this was offered.

It should be acknowledged that there are some limitations in the current literature on online therapy's effectiveness: it includes only a small number of randomised controlled trials and there is some inconsistent reporting of methodological features and results. So, we need more studies before we can say conclusively that online and phone therapy are as effective as in-person therapy, but the current evidence suggests that there is little difference. It's ultimately up to you, the client, and what you prefer and think will work best for you, in the context of your life.

To help with that decision, it's important to consider for yourself whether the practical benefits of online therapy outweigh seeing a therapist in person. The benefits include not having to travel and being able to slot therapy into your working day between other commitments. In terms of the therapy itself, you might be the sort of person who feels more comfortable in your own space. It's better that you begin therapy in a place where you feel safe and secure than you don't start at all. For the most socially anxious, if being seen is too difficult for you, there is the option of turning the video off. There can be some benefits to challenging those needs for safety, but you can do that in therapy once you've started, rather than forcing yourself into an uncomfortable situation that you might not manage to stick with.

There are some downsides to online therapy. It's important to take some time before and after sessions to plan for and look back on them. We spend so much of our lives running from one responsibility to another. Therapy is a space where you can take time for you; where you can slow down and think; where you can get in touch with how you are doing and what you are feeling. Online, there is the risk that you try to squeeze in sessions without carving out enough time for anything that emerges during the therapy to stick. What did you learn from the session? What are you taking away? What skills will you practise before the next session? Shutting down your video conferencing app and logging on immediately to your next work call is unlikely to be the best strategy for getting the most from your therapy.

Some downsides are logistical: the technology can break down from time to time, meaning you and your therapist will need a back-up plan if your internet connection drops. A good therapist these days needs to be confident in the basic essentials of using new technology, and it has to be said that, at the time of writing, a large percentage of therapists are not. You can spot that if you look at therapists' websites – some are clearly barely maintained; others are vibrant with posts and blogs and other up-to-date, relevant information. If you want to work online, make sure you choose a therapist who is tech savvy and has set up their technology properly so you can see and hear them clearly. Sarah Worley-James' guide (2022) is a useful reference for therapists and clients on how to work effectively online, across the range of media.

Phone-based therapy

A number of organisations offer 'affordable, convenient therapy' and a personalised service, matching you to the therapist who is most likely to help you with your specific problems. They promise to make the process simple and that you are free to change therapists if you don't like the one to whom you are assigned. They tell you they have thousands of therapists on their system, ready to help at any time of day or night. These organisations are global in their reach, of course, and position themselves at the heart of the internet revolution, pioneering the digitalisation of talking therapies.

The deal for you as a customer looks good: a month of therapy for about the usual price of a single session of in-person therapy. While these companies offer real-time video sessions and live messaging chat options with your therapist, their unique selling point, and the key technological development, is the ability for you as a client to exchange messages with your therapist via text, video or audio whenever you need to. You can come straight out of that difficult meeting with your boss or that argument with your partner and seek support from your therapist.

One of the traditional complaints about therapy, and we hear this from our own clients, is that you most need to speak with your therapist when you're most in need. You could do with speaking to them when you fear you're having a panic attack, or when your partner has just stormed off or threatened to dump you. You don't want to wait until your next booked session, when the impact might have worn off or you won't remember it so vividly.

This all sounds great, and is clearly popular: some of these companies claim to have more than a million users. It's already a big business. Businesses in the 'digital behavioural health' field raised $1.8 billion in venture-capital funding in 2020, up from $609 million in 2019 (Fischer, 2021).

However, the existing evidence doesn't tell a convincing story about the effectiveness of this therapy approach. One company's website quotes just one study (Marcelle et al., 2019) of 318 users of their platform, which claims to offer 'multimodal digital psychotherapy'. That study is itself carefully worded, saying only that it is a 'potentially' effective treatment for adult depression and that experimental trials are required before drawing a more conclusive finding.

The available research studies are small in size and don't tell a consistent story. One significant study (Goldberg et al., 2022), which brought together 14 meta-analyses of 145 randomised controlled trials and 47,940 participants, 'failed to find convincing evidence of efficacy' of digital therapy in all its formats (although there were some positive results for people seeking to stop smoking). There are also concerns about data privacy, given the lack of regulation in the sector (Fischer, 2021).

The Goldberg study suggests that digital therapy interventions *may* offer *some* hope for *some* reduction in anxiety and depression, although the effect sizes in the positive studies are generally small and the results rarely suggest that this type of therapy is any better than any other type of support such as behavioural activation (more exercise, better diet etc.). That might be enough to convince you, especially given the reduced cost compared with traditional therapy, but you might feel your mental health is valuable enough to spend more on better evidenced options.

Cost is clearly part of the explanation for why these services are popular, but it's not the only one. It's likely that any gains you make are due to factors that can be found in traditional therapy and not to the bolt-on extras you get online. Take, for example, the offer that you can change your therapist whenever you want. That's great when things are genuinely not working – for example, when the fit isn't right. We've discussed earlier in this book how the fit between you and your therapist is a major factor in therapy. However, another essential element of most good therapy is the need to be challenged and encouraged to step outside of your comfort zone. You might not want to go to that party because you feel too shy. You don't want to talk about the lack of sex in your relationship with your partner because it's too awkward. A good therapist will encourage you to 'lean in' to these issues where they are in line with your broader goals, even if that involves helping you confront your avoidance and your excuses. It might feel quite uncomfortable while they do so, and it probably should. Instead of changing your therapist at this point, or leaving therapy altogether, it's likely that you'd be better off meeting the challenge and pushing yourself, rather than giving in too quickly to the temptation to switch therapist when the going gets tough.

Similarly, having your therapist on call at all times, day or night, isn't always a positive. They can't, and shouldn't, be available 24 hours a day, seven days a week. Ultimately, you need to be able to live your own life, and that involves developing your own abilities to handle difficult issues, and that means exposure to difficult situations and learning to tolerate distress and make better decisions for yourself. You need to choose not to have that next drink, not to have someone always on hand to tell you not to.

Therapy is expensive for a reason. You wouldn't look for the cheapest solicitor if you were getting divorced, or the cheapest accountant to do your tax return. You want the reassurance that you're paying for someone who knows what they're doing. They're trained, they're regulated, they're professional. They keep on top of the latest research and continually update their skills. The best therapists use new technology to supplement your sessions – they can offer video sessions if your circumstances require it or together you agree it's therapeutically the best medium for you.

Virtual reality

Computer-generated simulations of reality, or 'virtual reality' (VR), offer excellent opportunities for good therapy, especially exposure-based approaches. Imagine you have a phobia of spiders (it's probably not that hard to imagine, given it is Britain's number one phobia (Manby, 2018)). A gradual exposure treatment for your phobia would usually start with looking at pictures of spiders until ultimately you can hold one of the scary critters. It's a well-evidenced approach to treating phobias (Wolitzky-Taylor et al., 2008), whether that's spiders, heights or crowded places. Being able to offer the option of handling and being around a VR spider seems like a useful tool in the therapist's toolkit. The therapist remains in control of the speed of exposure and can introduce necessary changes at a rate that is likely to be most useful for you.

The research supports the idea that VR is a useful tool in the therapist's kit, especially for managing phobias and for the treatment of post-traumatic stress disorder (for example, where a soldier is gradually exposed to similar computer-generated situations to the ones that caused their PTSD symptoms, while a therapist helps them with distress tolerance and regulation skills). One significant meta-analysis (Powers & Emmelkamp, 2008) found a large effect size for the use of VR exposure therapy in the treatment of anxiety disorders.

However, unsurprisingly, the evidence suggests that VR is less useful for the biggest mental health problems (and the ones you are most likely to be seeking help for), especially depression, anxiety and relationship issues. One review (Emmelkamp & Meyerbröker, 2021) found 'hardly any evidence' that VR therapy is effective in treating generalised anxiety disorder or obsessive-compulsive disorder. Another (Zeng et al., 2018) found that the current evidence was insufficient to support the advantages of VR therapy over traditional therapy for anxiety, depression or relationship issues, 'given the paucity of studies, small sample sizes, and lack of high-quality research designs'.

So, if you're suffering from a specific phobia or a traumatic response to a single event such as a car accident or a violent attack – the issues that CBT is generally recommended for – VR might be a useful part of your treatment when you're accompanied by a skilled and trained therapist. You might want proactively to seek out a therapist trained and experienced in using it, but you will probably want to ask how VR will be combined with other elements of an evidence-based exposure treatment plan. And if you are seeking therapy for problems such as stress, generalised anxiety and depression, the research suggests you're best off with traditional talking therapy.

Chatbots

Chatbots are everywhere in the modern economy. If you log on to your utility provider's website, a chatbot is likely to appear immediately and invite you to get in touch with your questions so they can direct you to the right support and, if you're lucky, to a human being who might be able to help. Although the primary aim is to save money, the best chatbots can be useful. They can provide a triage function, making sure you don't waste time having to explain your problem to numerous people before you are directed to someone who can actually help. Some chatbots very plausibly replicate human conversation in telephone interactions, as well as in text online.

When you ask a chatbot a question, it scans for words it recognises, and then gives you what it deems to be the most appropriate response from a set list. At the moment, these response lists are generally developed by humans, although artificial intelligence-generated chatbots such as ChatGPT will change the playing field in the next few years.

And mental health is no exception. Woebot, the American robotic therapist, offers expressions of empathy that can be very reassuring. There are also some very funny reports (Dinneen, 2020) of woeful and misattuned exchanges. But, given the scale of global mental health problems and the evidence behind the effectiveness of sometimes simple CBT interventions, it's worth paying attention to their development.

The most popular options specialise in simple CBT responses. That makes sense, as CBT works by challenging your thoughts and preventing catastrophic or black-and-white thinking. As we have seen elsewhere in this book, however, the success of CBT doesn't just depend on the specific techniques your therapist uses to help you challenge your thinking; it also depends on your fit and relationship with your therapist. Your therapist will also help you monitor your progress and will tailor their approach to your specific circumstances, including what you want to achieve in your life: your goals and aspirations. Despite the stereotype of CBT, it's rarely practised as a simple, standardised, worksheet-based treatment. Chatbots, in contrast, are limited when it comes to providing anything other than fairly basic responses, though this is likely to evolve very quickly in the years to come.

As Woebot exemplifies, chatbots can do it kindly and with seemingly genuine warmth and concern. But the evidence base in support of their effectiveness is almost non-existent. Research (Gilbody et al., 2015) into the effects of some popular CBT programmes using chatbots did not find any benefit over care as usual in primary care settings. In other words, the chatbots added nothing to the patient's likelihood of getting better. Save your money, or use it to better effect by buying an evidence-based CBT workbook to challenge your cognitive errors. A chatbot seemingly brings nothing additional to the process. And we refer you back to the evidence we cited in Chapter 4 that apps too are more effective if a real, live talking therapist is there to motivate and review your progress.

One area where simple, digital interventions *do* seem to help is via self-help versions of CBT where the treatment is delivered through a book or a computer programme. The treatment has been shown to give benefits in mild to moderate depression (Ridgway & Williams, 2011), in bulimia (Carrard et al., 2011), and in many, but not all, anxiety disorders (Kumar et al., 2017). It is a standardised intervention and can feel simplistic, but the evidence suggests it can help some people who need a little nudge in the right direction in terms of thinking more objectively or challenging their ways of seeing the world. It's also likely to be more readily available for free via your GP than treatments recommended by NICE.

Not all self-help digital interventions are good, though, so choose carefully. In a review (Sucala et al., 2017) of 52 apps for anxiety, an international team of psychologists found that 67% had been developed without any professional guidance from therapists or psychologists. In another review (Kertz et al., 2017), none of the 25 highest-rated apps for anxiety contained any content that was in line with the most up-to-date evidence-based treatments.

Summing it up

Therapy hasn't changed much in more than a century. That speaks to the core of what has made therapy so helpful to so many people, but also to a fundamental conservatism in a profession that fears and distrusts the new and the technological. But the use of technology in therapy is changing very fast. It's hard to predict the ways in which, for example, virtual reality and the metaverse will change the industry, but it seems very likely that developments in technology will produce therapists created by artificial intelligence that are capable of identifying in real time what is most likely to be the most therapeutic response for you and your specific mental health problems. Will they be as good as real therapeutic relationships? Will it matter to clients if their therapist feels human but isn't, so long as the end result is the same? Might some people – those who are very strongly averse to telling strangers their problems – actually prefer talking to a robot?

We don't know. But that day has not yet come. The evidence suggests that the best therapy for you still requires a well-trained therapist to meet with you, over several weeks at least, in person, on a screen or by phone. You still have to do the hard graft of making the changes you want in your life, and pay for them in most cases, in order to get the best fit. It will require money and hard work. How much is it worth to you to save your marriage, your career, your mental health? It's highly likely it will be worth that investment.

The speed of technological change in mental health is rapid. Similarly, the pace in the development of psychiatric drugs accelerated in the late twentieth century, powered by the 'chemical imbalance' hypothesis. Antidepressants proved helpful for many, but the hype exceeded their effectiveness, and minimised the side effects. So, what can psychiatry, medication and the re-emerging field of psychedelic-assisted therapy offer as an adjunct or alternative to the hard graft of therapy? We'll answer that question in the next chapter.

Ten things to remember

1. Use of information technology in therapy is already radically changing how therapists work and your relationship with your therapist. There are now many different ways for you to connect via your computer or smartphone.
2. Computer-based CBT might well be a good option to begin with. It's evidence-based and won't take up much time or money. It's easily available, and a good starting point from which to consider why you feel the way you do and what you can do to change that.
3. Online therapy seems to be as helpful as in-person therapy. Based on the evidence, it's for you to decide if its benefits outweigh the benefits of being in the same room as your therapist.
4. Bear in mind that many therapists who offer online options are offering it as a 'bolt on' to their in-person practice. Make sure they're competent at using the IT and have set it up properly.
5. Cheaper and more convenient online and digital options for therapy are emerging. However, the current evidence suggests that the genuinely new aspects of these services, such as being able to message your therapist any time of the day or night, don't add much to your likelihood of feeling better.
6. If you are tempted by the convenience and low cost of online subscription therapy services, remember that you might be doing yourself a disservice if you act like a consumer and change your therapist every time they challenge you or encourage you out of your comfort zone. Confronting those issues with a good therapist is often one of the most helpful things you can do in therapy.
7. Treatment options that incorporate virtual reality into their service are likely to be of help if you're suffering from something specific like a phobia or a single event trauma that responds to CBT techniques. However, it is unlikely to add much to your therapy if you're struggling with depression, stress or more general anxiety.
8. Chatbots are probably not helpful. The evidence is lacking. If cost is an issue, you're better off buying yourself an evidence-based therapy workbook.

9. However, keep an eye on options involving 'reinforcement learning' such as ChatGPT. They offer exciting opportunities for therapy interventions in the coming years and decades.
10. Good therapy requires investment: of your time, money and energy. If you've bought this book, it's likely that you think it is worth investing in your mental health. So, invest in the right therapy for you. There are no shortcuts.

Chapter 8
Medication and psychedelics

Can you improve your mental health without going to therapy? To an extent, yes. We know that eating well (Firth et al., 2019), improving your social support (Harandi et al., 2017) and sleeping well (Scott et al., 2021) are all likely to improve your mental health. So too are exercise and contributing to your community.

You'll notice, though, that none of those options is a magic-bullet solution. They all need a fair bit of consistency and application, and are habits that require a daily focus. You won't get better mental health by eating well for a week and then returning to the junk food. It won't help to go for an occasional walk or take out a gym membership and then never go more than once a month. It won't necessarily deal with other problems in your life, either – your lack of self-esteem, your inability to form sustaining relationships, your difficulties achieving your goals at work or in life generally, and so on.

In this chapter, we focus on two interventions that have, in their history, been sold as potential magic-bullet solutions to mental health problems: psychiatric medication and psychedelics, and especially the re-emerging field of psychedelic-assisted therapy.

In the first three months of 2022 in England, health services, especially GPs, prescribed 21 million antidepressant drugs, approximately double the number from a decade earlier (NHS Business Services Authority, 2022). Some blame GPs' readiness to prescribe, others the lack of better options, but the reality is that, for many, antidepressants are a big help in their journey to better mental health. For many, though, the rapid climb in antidepressant prescriptions signals something important about our society: that we are medicalising normal human responses to grief and stress, underfunding non-medical options such as therapy, and ignoring wider, structural changes that are required for our emotional health. These critics also point to the significant side effects and risk of relapse many experience when taking psychiatric medication.

Another approach that is fast gaining ground is psychedelic-assisted psychotherapy, which seems to offer a rapid route to insight, acceptance and symptom reduction.

This chapter guides you through the evidence for both.

Psychiatric medication

A psychiatric drug is one that has an effect on the chemical make-up of the brain and nervous system. The main types are antidepressants, antipsychotics, sleeping pills and tranquillisers (often called anti-anxiety medication). The vast majority of people who take psychiatric medication are seeking a quick fix to help reduce anxiety and/or depressive symptoms, so this is where we'll focus our attention.

We are not psychiatrists or medical doctors. You should consult your GP about medication if it feels like it might be the right choice for you or if you are already taking it and wondering if you have chosen wisely. What follows is an overview to help you understand your options.

Antidepressants

Depression is the most common mental health problem worldwide (Lim et al., 2018). Unsurprisingly, perhaps, antidepressant use is rising fast: the number of prescriptions in the UK doubled in the 10 years between 2008 and 2018 (Iacobucci, 2019).

A large part of the debate around the effectiveness of antidepressant medication has centred around beliefs and evidence about the causes of depression. It's been a longstanding, heated discussion between psychiatrists, psychologists and psychotherapists. Psychiatrists on the pro side quote research (Institute for Quality and Efficiency in Health Care, 2020) to show that antidepressants, and specifically SSRIs, achieve excellent results in treating low mood. The theory that underpins this side of the debate is that depression is caused by a chemical imbalance in the brain – specifically, low levels of the neurotransmitter serotonin. SSRIs block the brain's re-uptake of serotonin, and the resulting increased levels of serotonin seem to improve a person's low mood and help them either engage in therapy or get their life back on track.

On the 'against' or 'agnostic' side, psychologists and psychotherapists point to the evidence for the impact of real-world events (poverty, violence and abuse, relationship breakdown, poor housing and lack of opportunity) and internal struggles (lack of motivation, loneliness, low self-esteem) as causes for depression. They argue, on the basis of research, that the efficacy of medications has been greatly exaggerated and their harms minimised through flawed design and misreporting of trial data, some of which we covered in Chapter 4.

Research from a team at University College London (Moncrieff et al., 2022) seemed, at first glance, to settle the issue once and for all. The study was an umbrella review of studies over the last 50 years into the efficacy of SSRIs in treating depression. The review found no clear evidence that low serotonin levels cause depression. In addition, we know that antidepressants can cause serious side effects for some people, like nausea and insomnia, reduced sex drive, weight gain and withdrawal effects (Cartwright et al., 2016). They are also reported to cause emotional numbness. People can also spend years on these drugs, in the belief that they are taking some kind of maintenance dose. SSRIs weren't intended as such; they are supposed to effect recovery. The recommendation is to try them for six months and, if you decide with your doctor to go on taking them, review how you are getting on at six-monthly intervals (NICE, 2022). So, you'd be right to be careful when considering antidepressants, given the risks. But let's not forget that NICE recommends them because, in general, they are a helpful tool in treating low mood and anxiety-related conditions, including OCD, and the risk of side effects is sufficiently low for them to be included in its guidelines for treating a range of conditions.

Depression has, of course, much more complicated origins than simply an imbalance of a particular chemical in the brain. There is plentiful and incontrovertible evidence that depression is linked with events in people's lives. Richard Wilkinson and

Kate Pickett's books *The Spirit Level* (2009) and *The Inner Level* (2018) offer a comprehensive analysis of the relationship between adversity and depression. We have known for decades that SSRIs change serotonin levels pretty much immediately but take up to six weeks to make a difference to mood where they do have a positive effect (although the side effects kick in pretty much straight away). If depression was simply caused by serotonin levels, SSRIs would begin to improve mood levels within hours, not weeks.

So, low serotonin levels don't cause depression. But that doesn't mean antidepressants won't be helpful in treating your depression. What the Moncrieff research *did not* claim was that antidepressants do not work. Instead, the researchers examined the *specific ways* SSRIs are supposed to work: by reducing the 'reuptake' of serotonin in the brain, thereby increasing serotonin levels. Essentially, they put the final nail in the coffin of the 'serotonin hypothesis' – it is not a good explanation for depression, and certainly not a complete one. A better explanation is the 'biopsychosocial' model that acknowledges the biological, psychological and social causes of depression.

One classic metaphor is headaches. Scientists do not think that a lack of paracetamol *causes* headaches (lots of other things might be the cause, such as stress, dehydration, too much sunlight, alcohol withdrawal and so on). But if we take a paracetamol tablet when we have a headache, we then usually feel a reduction in pain. This does not of course show a link between lack of paracetamol and headaches. Similarly, you do not need to believe that low serotonin levels *cause* depression to believe that taking SSRIs can work to improve your mood.

It's certainly possible that some people have a specific kind of depression that is linked to, not necessarily *caused by*, changes in the serotonin system. Antidepressants affect a number of different pathways and receptors in the brain, so they help people with a range of different types of depression, only some of which are linked to the serotonin system. There is increasing evidence (Albert, 2019) to suggest that antidepressants act as a catalyst for neuroplasticity, creating more links between different areas of the brain and more activity in parts of the brain linked to depression, such as the hippocampus. It's possible, then, that antidepressants act like putting petrol in the empty tank of a car or rekindling the embers of a fading fire. They give your brain a necessary kickstart. SSRIs can also be effective in treating other symptoms and conditions, such as obsessive compulsive disorder (Skapinakis et al., 2016).

The current evidence suggests that a combination of antidepressants and therapy is the best plan for the treatment of moderate and severe depression (Cuijpers et al., 2020; NICE, 2022). The medication can help improve your mood and raise your motivation levels to a point where you can engage more proactively with your therapy, so it becomes a virtuous circle. It should be acknowledged, though, that medication is not recommended as a first step for treating mild to moderate depression (which is more common than more severe depression) (NICE, 2022). Although antidepressants can be helpful in treating depression, they should not be seen as a treatment that is going to provide a shortcut on your journey towards long-term, sustainable, good mental health. Nor should they be seen as a 'cure'; relapse is an ever-present possibility.

Anti-anxiety medication

However, there is good evidence for the efficacy of anti-anxiety drugs in treating generalised and acute anxiety (Craske et al., 2009).

But you need to be careful when considering anti-anxiety medication, and especially the class of drugs called benzodiazepines. You probably know them by their trade names, such as Xanax and Valium. They're sedatives, which increase the effects of something called gamma aminobutyric acid (GABA) in your system (Pritchett et al., 1989). GABA is a major inhibitory neurotransmitter. This means that GABA in a sense says 'stop it' to your brain and inhibits action: for example, slowing your automatic fear response. It allows the prefrontal cortex, the part of the brain behind your eyes that governs executive control, more time to get back in the driver's seat. Another positive of benzodiazepines is that, unlike SSRIs, they work very quickly, relaxing your muscles and mind within hours.

That all sounds great. But benzodiazepines are likely to make you feel sleepy and drowsy, which is not good for day-to-day functioning. You wouldn't use them for normal life distress either, such as dealing with understandable grief following a significant death or divorce. Most importantly, they have a strong addictive quality, which means your GP should not prescribe them for anything other than an immediate crisis, and for just a few weeks at most, and not above a very low dose.

Beta blockers are an alternative medication option for anxiety, but only for specific short-term situations where you face acute physical anxiety symptoms: for example, you have a phobia of public speaking or flying on a plane, or you have to take an important exam. They're not actually psychiatric medication, in that they treat the physical but not the psychological symptoms of anxiety. So they are not a good option for more generalised anxiety and stress in life.

Your best medication option for anxiety, alongside good therapy, is an SSRI such as citalopram (Strawn et al., 2018). You may find that surprising, given that SSRIs are generally considered to be antidepressants. However, NICE recommends them for generalised anxiety (NICE, 2011). Taking an SSRI does not necessarily mean you have depression.

Psychedelic-assisted therapy

Psychedelic-assisted therapy has emerged quite recently as a possible silver-bullet solution to tackling serious and seemingly unshifting depression. It would be more exact to say re-emerged, as there was considerable work done in the 1960s into use of psychedelic substances for mental health problems, which was stopped in its tracks by the crackdown on these drugs to control their recreational use. Since then, its advocates have persistently continued to research their use and seem slowly to be gaining ground in terms of amassing the necessary evidence for efficacy required to convince the drug regulatory authorities to allow their prescription as a medical treatment.

You've probably heard these psychedelic substances referred to as hallucinogens. Put simply, they're substances that create changes in your brain that alter your perceptions: what you see, how you feel, how you think. A lot of what you see or hear while taking psychedelics doesn't exist: your brain is creating those images and sounds inside your head. Some people describe the experience of taking hallucinogens as being similar to losing their sense of self. This is experienced mainly in a positive way, but potentially can be very disorientating.

Some psychedelics are found naturally, such as psilocybin (magic mushrooms), ayahuasca (a drink brewed from various South American plants), and peyote, which is a psychedelic cactus. LSD is made from a substance found in a fungus. Other psychedelics are synthetic drugs made in laboratories. The most commonly known is MDMA, or 3,4-Methylenedioxymethamphetamine, to use its full name. You probably know it as Ecstasy. It's a stimulant as well as a hallucinogen. Then there's ketamine, which is licensed for medical use in the UK. It is known as a 'dissociative anaesthetic', and is safer to use with children and vulnerable older people. But it is already widely used also as a treatment for depression, for pain management, and as a recreational drug.

In psychedelic-assisted *therapy*, psychedelics are used in combination with talking therapy. Its proponents are very clear that this is a package: the benefits of the psychedelic in releasing people's brains from being locked into certain ways of thinking and seeing the world cannot be sustained without the talking therapy to consolidate and build on the opportunities it offers for people to change their thought patterns. There have been some very exciting early studies into its effectiveness (see Nutt, 2019; Nutt et al., 2020). This type of therapy seems to offer hope for deeply entrenched conditions like constantly recurring depression and addictions. For example, a study (Bogenschutz et al., 2022) has found that therapy facilitated by psilocybin significantly reduces heavy drinking in those struggling with alcohol abuse, and there are others showing promise for a range of psychiatric disorders (da Costa et al., 2022).

A key benefit is the speed of change and lasting benefits. The therapy itself is intensive – at least three or four five-hour sessions of drug treatment, and nine more intensive one-hour therapy sessions before and after the drug is used to prepare the patient and reinforce its benefits. Some of the first-person anecdotal evidence accompanying some of these trials is very powerful, too. In a BBC documentary, a participant who had psilocybin-assisted therapy said, 'Talking therapy helps you believe something to be true. Psilocybin helps you *know* it' (cited in Eastal, 2021). Others talk of the experience as being like a ski slope: the patient has spent all their life stuck in the same tracks. Taking the drug is like a heavy fall of snow: suddenly a vast vista of untrammelled slope opens up, offering them the chance to go fearlessly in any direction. Here is where the skilled guidance of the therapist, with specialist training, is considered vital (Jackson, 2023).

An additional benefit is that there seem to be relatively few side effects from the psychedelics, or risks of overdose, compared with antidepressants. For the classic psychedelics like psilocybin and LSD, there is a minimal to zero risk of addiction. That's not the case with anti-anxiety medication like benzodiazepines. However, there are some potentially worrying health risks that do need to be watched for: recreational use of psychedelics can trigger psychotic or manic episodes in people with history of schizophrenia or bipolar disorder. Psilocybin and ketamine raise blood pressure and heart rate, so those with heart conditions, high blood pressure and arrhythmias are advised not to take them. And one trial (COMPASS Pathways, 2022) of psilocybin showed a number of patients experiencing serious side effects, such as suicidal thoughts and behaviour, and these increased as the dose increased. This is in part why the therapists involved need specialist training, to ensure the substances are used safely as well as effectively.

Things are moving quickly from trials to clinical treatment. Ketamine-assisted therapy clinics are now open in the UK (BBC News, 2021). And a psychedelics industry is already flourishing, with more than 80 companies investing in developing and administering psychedelic compounds for mental health treatment, and big claims being made about the effectiveness of psychedelic-assisted therapy (Halford, 2022).

There is an attractive and understandable mystical appeal to psychedelics. They offer a unique opportunity for us to delve below the conscious mind to discover what lies within. They even offer the prospect of therapy being an enjoyable voyage of discovery. If we can discover successful treatments that can go to the heart of our inner distress without the investment of time, energy, stress, pain and money involved in much successful therapy, we would want people to access them.

However, it's best to stay cautious, given the state of the research into psychedelic-assisted therapy. As with the research base for psychiatric drugs, the researchers involved in these pioneering studies are, in some cases, being paid by the companies looking to reap rich rewards from this promising sector. The field itself is still small, limiting the pool of peer reviewers of papers submitted for publication. And much of the media reporting on the research focuses on the encouraging results, and typically says little to nothing about less favourable findings. For example, psilocybin outcomes in treating depression in one major study were treated in the media as being revolutionary, but were only as statistically significant as the antidepressant they were being compared with in the study (Ritchie, 2022).

So, in short, to prove its efficacy, psychedelic-assisted therapy needs many more, bigger, peer-reviewed studies that are independent of any commercial interest. But it will be exciting to see where the research takes us in the years to come.

And, bringing us back to the subject of this book, the effectiveness of psychedelic therapy is thought to depend on a complex group of interlocking factors, and is not limited to the psychedelic compound. Psychedelics are not a magic bullet either. Other factors thought to contribute to the therapy's success include patient expectations (the belief that the treatment is going to work), the environment in which it's performed (does it feel calming and safe?) and the strength of the relationship with the therapist (are they able to guide you to build on and apply your insights?). These are consistent with what we know makes good therapy. The therapy element of psychedelic-assisted therapy could be seen to be as crucial, if not more crucial, than the compound itself.

Summing it up

There is strong evidence that medication, especially SSRIs, can be a helpful tool for many for managing their depression and anxiety, especially for defined periods and in combination with other interventions, such as good psychotherapy. But on their own, they're not a silver-bullet treatment, and for more common problems, such as mild to moderate depression, they are not recommended for first-line use.

We also know that there are some significant potential benefits from psychedelic-assisted therapy, as well as some potential harms. But at present, the research base is not rich or deep enough to be able to say it can achieve benefits where so many other available treatments have failed.

It's understandable that you would want a quick fix, especially if it's a pleasant fix. The prospect of a simple, lasting solution to all of life's problems – your relationship problems, your addictions, your depression, your anxiety – is attractive. But the simple fact remains that you will at some point have to confront those challenging psychological problems and do life differently. Effective therapy is about confrontation and change, not avoidance. And as we've made clear at every point in this book, effort matters. There are no silver bullets and meaningful change is hard won and requires effort, resolve and persistent.

So, knowing there's no quick fix or magic pill to fix your mental health struggles, the question is: are you serious and ready to take the plunge and start therapy? We'll help you out in our final chapter.

Ten things to remember

1. Psychiatric medication and psychedelic-assisted therapy offer alternatives to the hard work of therapy. But neither are magic bullets. The evidence base for the former is hotly contested, and research is still in its infancy for the latter.
2. If you think psychiatric medication like antidepressants might help you, your starting point should be to talk to your GP or a psychiatrist. Ask lots of questions and take your time before beginning medication treatment.
3. While we don't know exactly what causes depression, we do have evidence that SSRIs are beneficial for a lot of people with moderate and severe depression. They should not be used for milder kinds of depression, where therapy is your best option.
4. SSRIs are likely your best medication option if you suffer from generalised anxiety or obsessive-compulsive disorder.
5. The most common medications come with significant risks, despite their potential benefits, such as reduced sex drive, blunted emotions and weight gain. Make sure you find out about and weigh up the potential benefits and risks before you start taking them.

6. If you do suffer side effects, contact your GP immediately. You can change medication or taper off your medication over time.
7. These drugs are not intended for lifetime use. Regularly review their effectiveness if your doctor keeps prescribing them for longer than six months. If they don't help after six months, you may want to look for an alternative.
8. The research on psychedelic-assisted therapy is incredibly exciting. It might become a major tool for treating severe and intractable mental health problems, especially trauma-related conditions, addictions and depression, over the next few decades.
9. However, the research is in its very early stages, and most of these substances are not legal in most Western countries, not even for medical use. So, the jury remains out. Watch the space.
10. It's tempting to think you can hack your way to better mental health. But the deep changes needed in many cases can't be hacked. Find yourself a good therapist and put in the hard graft, alongside medication if it helps. It will take all of this to make your life better.

Chapter 9
Are you ready and are you serious?

Good therapy and a good therapist are critical to getting a good outcome from therapy. But, ultimately, what matters most is your motivation and the effort you put into the process. Our final chapter asks you to honestly assess whether you are serious about changing and ready to do it.

It's the factors you bring into therapy, not your therapist or their techniques, that make up most of the difference in terms of how well therapy works. Research (Lambert, 2013) shows that 15% of the positive outcomes in therapy are down to therapist technique, 15% to your hopes and expectations, 30% to the relationship with your therapist and 40% to the so-called client factors – that is, what you bring with you to therapy. They include your background and history, interpersonal skills, motivation and social support, as well the problem or issue you are dealing with. In other words, it's you that makes the most difference.

This ought not to be a great surprise. In every field of human endeavour, effort counts. You get out what you put in. This can be seen in the research on peak performance (Ericsson et al., 2007) and the well-known idea that you need 10,000 hours of practice before you can excel at something. That idea is too simplistic on its own (Bradley, 2012), as both the author credited with making it popular (Gladwell, cited in Ericsson & Pool, 2016) and the original researchers have pointed out. But the basic notion still stands: the harder we try and the more we care about something, the more likely we are to succeed at it.

Therapy is no different. If you turn up late, aren't honest about what you're feeling and constantly blame others for your own situation, you won't get much out of it. So, in the first part of this chapter, we look at what you need to bring to therapy: a readiness to be honest about your own part in your problem and a willingness to do things differently, for example. The good news is you don't have to be anything like perfect or 100% ready to change. There are stages on the journey to change and we look at how therapy can help at each of those stages. But, ultimately, you need to take action if you are going to change your life. So, in the final part of the chapter, we provide a questionnaire to help you assess whether you are ready to start therapy.

Attitudes, attributes and habits

Habits form slowly and therefore change slowly

Perhaps the most important thing we know about behaviour change is that it isn't easy and it takes time. Changing your behaviour is seriously hard. When you come to therapy, you are often trying to change the ingrained habits of a lifetime, learned in childhood and practised over many years. Even when we assume someone has had a radical 'overnight' experience of change, that's rarely the case. Behind the scenes, that person came to see over time that their life was a mess, that their habits were costing them dearly and that they were hurting the people around them (Miller & Rose, 2009).

For example, most alcoholics have tried to stop drinking many times before finally being able to do so. And sobriety itself is usually a series of small steps, taken one day at a time. It's seldom if ever a heroic, solo, one-off effort of will power.

When you try to convince yourself that you are 100% ready for change, that it will be easy and that you can do it all at once, you set yourself ambitious goals. But that's more like wishful thinking than a realistic plan. As a consequence, you fail. Much better if you accept that behaviour is formed gradually over time, and therefore takes time and perseverance to change.

Focus on the smallest changes first

On the basis that habit change is hard, one of the best ideas is that 'little and often' works better than 'dramatic and bold'. This is the basic idea contained in James Clear's best-seller *Atomic Habits*

(Clear, 2018). The word 'atomic' refers here to doing something very small, but it also evokes the idea of immense energy and power contained in the other meaning of the word. The message of the book is that small, consistent actions create powerful impacts and generate impressive results.

This probably isn't the way you typically think about habits. Instead, maybe you tell yourself that you're going to get up and go to the gym before work, five days a week. The problem is you won't. Or you'll manage it for a week or two, then fail, tell yourself how useless you are and give up altogether. Really what you're saying when you make such grand 'all-or-nothing' plans is that, if you can't change immediately, all at once and without any effort or setbacks, then you can't be bothered.

Success is much more likely when you keep your plans achievable and simple. You are much better off going to the gym two or three times a week, at a convenient time that fits your schedule, and keeping that routine going for months and years. Small changes may seem insignificant, but they are not. In aviation, pilots know that, for every one degree they are off course, 60 miles further on, they will end up being one mile wide of their route. On a 14-hour flight, that's the difference between landing at your destination or running out of fuel over the Atlantic.

Be realistic, be prepared, create incentives and accountability

Generally, we are far too confident about how easy it will be to change. Such optimism is unhelpful. What you need is realism. The future version of you is no more self-disciplined than the current version of you. If you don't want to do it today, and you didn't do it yesterday, the chances are you won't do it tomorrow either. You need to learn from past failures, not wish them away. Change needs to be approached with realism, using strategy and skill.

The secret to a better life is not to eradicate the impulses that make us human (Milkman, 2021). Resisting sweet or calorific foods is difficult because eating this type of food in particular is a hard-wired, evolutionary impulse (Ramirez, 1990). That's the reason why self-help books with the simple message to 'just do it' don't work. Whether it's more exercise, eating less or anything else, relying on willpower alone is not enough for most people (Baumeister & Tierney, 2012). You need a strategy. It's much more likely you'll avoid sugary snacks if you've got healthy alternatives to hand. You are much more likely to eat fruit if it's there at hand when you walk into the kitchen, or in a bowl on your desk.

The trick is to make life easier for yourself. Research (Harris-Fry, 2017) shows that people who joined a gym less than four miles away went more than five times a month, whereas those who travelled five miles or more only went once a month. That one mile made a huge difference.

Or, to continue with the same example, maybe you need a personal trainer to come to your home. Often, we need to add a layer of accountability if we are to do things that are good for us but that we know we won't want to do. This is particularly true when first changing habits. Left to your own devices, you may well hit the snooze button and tell yourself that you'll go to the gym later or you'll do a double session tomorrow. You won't. But if the personal trainer is at your door or is expecting you to fetch up at 6.30am at the gym, the chances are you'll get up, however reluctantly. The same principle applies to therapy: having a regular slot and knowing you will have to pay up whether you go or not (barring illness or an emergency) makes you more likely to attend when you don't necessarily want to.

That said, ideally you're looking to enjoy your new-found habits. If you really hate the gym, you're probably not going to form a habit of going long term. In this case, you'd be better off trying walking, or swimming perhaps. The best exercise is not the one that burns the most calories, it's the one that you'll do on a repeat basis. But if you really can't find anything you like, try to find a way to 'sugar the pill'. One researcher (Milkman, 2021) suggests listening to your favourite podcast or current audiobook *only* when working out. If you can find ways to add rewards to things you don't particularly enjoy, then the release of dopamine in your brain will tie both together. And you are much more likely to stick to behaviours when they are accompanied by rewards.

Tailor your plans

Whether it's finding incentives, improving accountability or linking habits to rewards, what we're really talking about is tailoring strategies so that they work for you. That's one of the things that makes the most difference, according to recent thinking on behavioural change (Milkman, 2021). What works for someone else will not necessarily work for you. Goal setting, visualising success, linking activities to rewards and focusing on the smallest change first are all good ideas. They are based on research. But if they don't work for you, find something else that does.

That's the problem with simplistic messages like 'just do it'; they don't factor in the stage of change you are at or what works for you as an individual. Those messages assume that everyone starts from the same place and that all you need is sufficient willpower. But that's not borne out by research (Eyal, 2016). Wishing you ate better, drank less or exercised more will not alone make any difference to those habits. Telling yourself to 'own your problems', 'just do it', or 'master your mind' won't work either. You need to link your intentions to a strategy and plan that is tailored to you and takes into account the particular challenges you face (Milkman, 2021).

And that's where therapy can be helpful. Rather than going it alone, you can use therapy to help you connect to the values or purpose behind the change. Your therapist can also challenge your plans and stress-test your assumptions. Therapy can provide accountability too. Did the plan you put in place work, or does it need amending? Is it the right plan but do you need to put more effort in to make it work? It's easy to get lost or discouraged when you go it alone. Therapy can help you keep perspective, acknowledge progress, normalise setbacks and focus on doing the next right thing. In therapy, you can take realistic stock of what you're up against, whether that is the habits of a lifetime, evolutionary impulses, or deeply entrenched behaviours and ways of thinking. Therapy can help you take the challenge of change seriously.

The one non-negotiable

Although strategies and plans have to be tailored to you, there is one non-negotiable when it comes to change: you must believe that you can change (Eubanks & Goldfried, 2019). It's useful to be realistic and to know that change is difficult, but you have to believe that it's possible. You need at least a seed of hope. It can be watered and tended in therapy, but without that seed, nothing can grow.

Therapy is a fresh start and one of the best ways to generate change is to embrace the power of a fresh start (Milkman, cited in Geller, 2014). That's why people are so keen to make changes around the turn of the year. Sure, a lot of people fail in those resolutions when attempting them on their own – as many as 80%, by some estimates (Norcross, 2012) – but that still means 20% of the goals people set each year are met. And that's a lot of people who've changed their life for the better. The truth is that change is difficult but it's not impossible. If you come to therapy knowing change won't be easy, it will help you create an effective plan, put in the necessary work and ensure you don't get overwhelmed by setbacks.

The growth mindset and the need for grit

To put that another way, you have to adopt a 'growth mindset' for change to occur. Research in this area suggests that individuals who believe their talents and attributes can be developed through hard work, good strategies and help from others have a growth mindset (O'Keefe et al., 2018). They tend to achieve more than those who believe their attributes are fixed or innate. People with a growth mindset believe in change. They worry less about doing things perfectly and they put their energy into learning from mistakes and trying again.

This idea is linked to the notion of 'grit', another simple but important idea that emphasises the need for perseverance. The original research (Duckworth et al., 2007) in the United States suggested that grit is not only the single trait most likely to account for success but is also a better predictor of success than IQ.

Both ideas have been oversold as the answer to everything, as their originators have acknowledged (Dweck, 2018; Duckworth, cited in Kamenetz, 2016). Nevertheless, those simple ideas contain important truths. And both ideas link to the more fundamental and far-reaching notion of brain plasticity. Recent advances in neuroscience have shown that the brain is far more malleable than we used to think. We now know that, from the time our brain begins to develop, even before birth, until the time we die, the connections among the cells reorganise in response to our changing needs. Connectivity between neurons changes to allow us to learn and adapt to different experiences (Owens & Tanner, 2017).

While the brain is not actually a muscle, it operates a lot *like* a muscle. Physiological changes in the brain happen as the result of interactions with our environment as neural networks grow new connections or strengthen and speed up existing ones (Tierney & Nelson III, 2009). These fairly recent neuroscientific discoveries have shown us that we can increase our neural growth via the habits we develop. The ability of the brain to reorganise and reform synaptic connections in response to learning or experience is one of the most important discoveries in neurobiology, with profound implications for personal change and growth. Some writers (Jarrett, 2021) have used this and similar ideas to highlight the fact that we can change in profound and radical ways not previously thought possible.

Sometimes you need to heal first, before you can change and grow

So, you need perseverance and a belief that change is possible in order to change. And the good news is that neuroscience is on your side. But, let's be honest, most people don't arrive at therapy full of determination to change and grow. Often you arrive feeling stuck, broken or lost. That's fine too. Change takes place in stages, as we will see below.

This point is often missing from self-help books with compelling messages of encouragement or instruction. Sometimes you need to rebuild or heal first. In this case, therapy, uniquely, can help with the change process. Good therapy allows you to make sense of difficult experiences. A good therapist will validate and normalise your problems and help you see why you struggle as you do. If you have grown up having your confidence undermined or if you have suffered more severe forms of neglect or abuse, this will have had a profound effect on you. The person you have become reflects your underlying neural architecture, which has been shaped by many years of experience.

Our earliest attachments provide templates for our subsequent relationships. As a result of that, we repeat relationship patterns throughout our lives. Because we've lived with them for all of our lives, they are more or less invisible to us. That's why you can't just *decide* to be different. The message to 'just do it' ignores the fact that often you don't know how to spot, let alone solve, your own problems. Even when you know what you *should* be doing, you can't just do it, and that's the reason you come to therapy.

In therapy, you come to see that your problems – never feeling quite good enough or being excessively self-critical – are not your fault. They are often rooted in your early experiences of home, school and friendship. In therapy, you become aware that you find certain situations difficult and are therefore less likely to be blindsided by them in future. You learn to pause and evaluate feelings. Is your mind running at 100mph, imagining the worst-case scenario? Can you pause and take a more realistic view? Or can you accept your feelings, without acting on them, knowing they will pass? Good therapy is absolutely about taking ownership of your problems and taking action to improve your life, but with skill and compassion and at a pace that is right for you.

Putting it all together

Motivation comes and goes. The question is not, 'How do I avoid dips in motivation?' but, 'How do I respond when dips inevitably happen?' And it turns out that you can *do* what matters, even if you don't *feel* much like it, especially if you keep focused on the meaning, purpose or values behind your actions.

This idea of the importance of values and purpose to guide effort shows up in sports psychology in particular. Repetition, drudgery and pain are often essential to success and need to be sustained by dreams, goals or commitment to team mates: i.e. the meaning and purpose behind the effort.

In sports and other performance settings, the importance of *aiming*, *sustaining* and then *regaining* your attention is also central (Mumford, 2015). Having put your attention where you want it – on the activity or outcome, not the crowd or how much your muscles are hurting – you then need to keep it there. Inevitably your mind will wander. You'll think of reasons not to bother, or you'll be distracted by what's going on around you. At that point, you need to regain your attention in the shortest time possible. Tuning into values, purpose and meaning is one way to do so. This moment-by-moment mindful awareness of returning your attention where you want it to be is an ongoing challenge in life, as well as in sports.

We should also say, useful though it is, mindfulness is another idea that has been oversold as the answer to everything (Purser, 2019). In many settings, it simply doesn't work, as has been clearly shown by a recent large-scale study (Kuyken et al., 2022) in schools, where being taught mindfulness had no impact on preventing mental health problems or promoting wellbeing among pupils (the researchers concluded that many pupils found it boring and therefore didn't practise it at home). Nevertheless, if you are serious about making the time to practise, moment by moment awareness of your attention is usually a critical component of performance (Mumford, 2015), of change (Milkman, 2021), of living a good life more generally (Kabat-Zinn, 2013) and of making the most of therapy (Wallin, 2007). This is confirmed by decades of studies (Davidson & Lutz, 2008) showing that meditation alters the very structure and function of the brain.

In summary, there is no way around this kind of focus and effort. It doesn't matter how good a therapist you choose, they can't do the work for you. They can help you formulate a strategy tailored to you, but *you* have to follow it. You are in therapy for 50 minutes a week. There are 167 hours remaining in the week when you are on your own. If you're not focusing your attention or using your values to drive you on and keep you going on the darker days, you are not going to change.

Five stages of change

Having considered some of the most fundamental and enduring principles of change and how they apply to therapy, let's look at the *stages* of change that researchers have identified and see where you are in terms of being ready to begin the hard work of improving your life.

One of the best known frameworks (Prochaska & DiClemente, 1986) for thinking about change describes five distinct stages. The authors of the framework say that this framework applies even across quite different problems or goals. Let's consider each of those stages, and how therapy can help.

1. Pre-contemplation

At this stage, you have little or no intention of changing your behaviour in the near future. Family and friends might see the problem, but you don't. Without any motivation to change, you are very unlikely to do so. Change is hard: you need a strong incentive and willingness to work at it. At this stage, a conversation with even the most brilliant therapist is likely to be a waste of time and money.

2. Contemplation

At this stage, you are aware that a problem exists and you are thinking seriously about it, but you have not yet made a commitment to take any action. You start to think that perhaps you should act differently, and to count the cost of your actions. But you're not sure that you can really improve things. Or perhaps you worry that you've tried and failed before, or that you don't know where to begin. This stage can be an unhappy place if you stay here too long, focused on your problems but not yet doing anything about them. Lots of people come to therapy at this stage and it can sharpen your focus on the cost of your behaviour (physical/emotional/financial), as well as the benefit of changing to you and the people around you.

3. Preparation

The next stage is made up of good intentions or small actions. You know you need to get things sorted but you haven't yet taken the kind of significant action that would resolve the problem. The questions at this stage become, how are you actually going to do this, and how will this time be different from other times? Therapy can help you work out *what exactly you want to do differently, how you will go about it and the effort you are prepared to put in.* A lot of people rush straight to action, only to find they don't have a sufficiently robust plan. Therapy helps you prepare properly so that you save yourself time and effort in the long run, just as you would prepare for any important journey.

4. Action

This is the stage when you start to change your behaviour and do something differently. This stage requires considerable commitment, effort and persistence. Even when you know your goals and you're clear that you want to change your behaviour, it's still normal to return to old habits: they are familiar and comfortable and it's often scary to do things differently. You need to accept that there will likely be slips, trips and falls along the way. Therapy can help you stay the course, come to terms with the fact that change isn't easy, and make sure you don't beat yourself up over inevitable setbacks. As well as providing accountability and encouragement, therapy can also help you decide what's working and adjust your strategy or increase the amount of effort needed.

5. Maintenance

In the final stage of the change process, you are seeking to prevent a relapse and trying to consolidate your gains. Getting started is only half the battle; the other half is sticking with it and turning new behaviours into habits. Often that means doing things when you don't feel like it. In many ways, this is the most important phase of change. Therapy offers additional accountability, feedback and support at this stage, in much the same way that athletes or performers work with coaches or teachers to maintain their performance. You might be tempted to think you can 'go it alone'. That's often a mistake. Many people can kickstart a change, but far fewer can maintain it. Take this stage seriously and stack the odds of longer-term change in your favour by building in help.

Summing up the stages of change

First you need to recognise the things you want to change; then you need to weigh up the effort needed and decide if it's worth it. If it is, you need to work out the best way of making those changes. Then you need to get going by taking action and flexing your strategy, depending on how successful it is. Finally, you need to keep going when it's difficult, bounce back if you slip up, and lock those changes into new habits and a new way of life. Easy to say; difficult to do.

One of the most reliable ways of making those changes stick is to recognise where you are in the stages of change, and to work through them in a methodical way. In one study, two identical groups were followed and those who worked through each of the stages were 10 times more successful than those who did not. That same study found that each step you take nearly doubles the probability of your long-term success (Norcross, 2012). The researchers behind the work sum that up by saying that it's about doing the right thing at the right time.

The other way of summarising the advice above is to say that it highlights the importance of personalising the way you approach change, in line with where you are in the stages of change. Sometimes you know exactly what you want (to stop drinking, for example), and you are ready to take action. But other times you don't know what you want, you just know something is wrong (for example, life has lost its meaning since the breakdown of your relationship). If you know what you want, you can move to preparing for action and then get straight on with it. But if you don't yet know what you want, you'll need to start further back, and therapy can help you work out what you want, how you'll go about it, and whether you're prepared to put in the effort.

The Readiness for Therapy questionnaire

Now you know where you are in terms of the stages of change, let's get practical and see if you are ready to start therapy by considering the questions contained in the Readiness for Therapy Questionnaire (RTQ) (Ghomi et al., 2020).

The RTQ was created by researchers following a review of the literature and interviews with hundreds of clients after therapy. The researchers' objective was to create a set of questions that would predict how well clients would do in therapy (measured by comparing how they described their problems before and after therapy). For years, being ready for change has been an important part of assessing suitability for therapy. But now we have a tool that reliably predicts this. By answering a few simple questions, you can now anticipate whether you are likely to have a positive outcome from therapy.

As you consider the questions below, bear in mind that there are no wrong answers: *you are where you are* in terms of readiness for change. It is better to know that than pretend you are further forward. So, answer the questions honestly. They are simple and direct, but they are revealing precisely because they are the kinds of questions we often try to avoid.

Also note that there is no single cut-off point and you won't be given an overall numerical score when you've completed the questionnaire. Your answers will give you a strong indication of whether therapy is likely to be the right choice for you, but they will not say absolutely whether you are ready or not. That is still for you to decide, of course.

With that in mind, ask yourself the following six questions and decide whether you strongly agree, agree, are undecided, disagree or strongly disagree.

1. It is essential that I work on my problems as soon as possible because they are affecting the quality of my life.
2. I like to do things the way I've always done them, and I don't want to change.
3. If I'm sceptical about something, I am not willing to try.
4. Even if therapy becomes difficult, I will stick with it.
5. In between sessions, I will dedicate time to practising regularly the things I have learned in therapy.
6. I won't attend therapy if I have something more pressing or interesting planned.

If you've answered mainly that you 'agree' or 'strongly agree' to statements 1, 4 and 5, and mainly 'disagree' or 'strongly disagree' with statements 2, 3 and 6, then you are probably well placed to benefit from therapy. If not, that may indicate that you are not yet ready. You can always return to the questions at a later date.

For the most part, we'd guess that if you have read this far and taken the time to complete the questionnaire, your answers probably indicate that you would benefit from therapy. That doesn't mean complete and total agreement with every statement. Maybe you would be tempted to cancel at the last minute or you feel a bit reluctant to practise between sessions. That's useful information. You now know you have that tendency; it doesn't mean you have to act on it. Very few people are in 100% agreement with all those statements or completely committed to change. Yet, as we pointed out at the very start of this book, 76% of people who have had therapy say they would recommend it to a friend or family member (BACP, 2019).

But I still can't find the time or money

Maybe you still think you can't find the time. Sure, therapy takes time, but be honest with yourself: therapy typically will take up just 50 minutes of your week. Many therapists will see you online, eliminating travel time (online therapy works just as well as more traditional in-person therapy, as discussed in Chapter 7).

Or perhaps you are telling yourself that your problems are so serious that they will take years to resolve. That may be the case, but usually it's not so. Knowing exactly how long therapy will take is a bit like knowing how long a piece of string is. But what we do know is that lots of problems can be resolved, or significantly improved, in just weeks or months; it need not take years (Layard & Clark, 2015a). Sometimes, surprisingly, they can be resolved in a single session (Dryden, 2019).

Nevertheless, some issues do require more time, among them eating disorders, addictions and what is sometimes called complicated childhood trauma. But they are the exceptions, not the rule. And even in those instances, you can pause or stop along the way. Therapy is similar to getting physically fit: the ultimate goal might be a complete fitness overhaul, but you will progress in stages – losing weight, increasing muscle mass and improving oxygen consumption – all of which have an impact on life expectancy. So, you may have stopped short of your stated goals, but what you have achieved may still be life changing. The same is true in therapy.

Maybe money feels like the barrier. Private therapy is expensive and it's out of reach for many people. If you are in that position and you have exhausted everything offered by the NHS (including self-referral to online help), you may be able to access low-cost therapy via a local or national charity. You will most likely have to wait, and you may be seen by a student in training, but don't immediately be put off by this. That person will be working with only a small number of clients and will be carefully supervised by a much more experienced therapist. If money is the issue, it is well worth considering this as an option.

If you can afford it, the cost of therapy is comparable with the cost of a haircut, massage or osteopathy. Expensive though it is, a lot of good therapy can be found for about the same price as a coffee, croissant and sandwich each day for a week. Or you could think of it as the same cost as a decent meal for two.

It's worth considering the consequences of not getting help, too. What does your current problem cost you and what would you gain from the change? Maybe it takes a toll on your health and fitness. Or maybe there is a cost in terms of your performance at work. Or perhaps the impact is closer to home – on children, family and friends, or on your partner.

As we have emphasised in this chapter, change will be hard and it comes at a cost. But for most people, most of the time, with most problems, therapy is a shrewd investment of time and money.

Summing it up

Although outcomes aren't guaranteed, three-quarters of people benefit from therapy and say they would recommend it (BACP, 2019). If you follow the suggestions and prompts in this book, it's likely you will have the same positive experience too.

Of course, that does mean that not everybody benefits, as we have seen. NHS statistics (NHS Digital, 2021) make this very point: lots of people stop coming to therapy. Some stop because they have got what they needed. This finding (Dryden, 2019) shows up again and again in research. But others stop because they didn't find it helpful. Therapy is a lot like other interventions in medicine and healthcare: there are no guarantees and they don't always work. But, as we've seen, there are lots of things you can do to reduce that risk.

If you're clear about your preferences for the type of therapy and therapist that will suit you, and if you know where you are in the change cycle, then you significantly increase your chances of getting good outcomes from therapy. Combined with your willingness to work hard, by far the most likely outcome is significant improvement within a relatively short period of time.

So, be honest about where you are, recognise that therapy will be hard work, but get started. If you keep turning up, keep being honest, keep taking responsibility and keep taking a risk on doing things differently, therapy is likely to change your life for the better.

If you've read this far, it's time to take action now. Use the chapter summaries to remind yourself of the most important points when selecting a type of therapy and a therapist, consider just how much your problems are costing you at present, remember that you are more resilient than you think you are, summon up your courage, and go and get yourself some life-changing therapy.

Ten things to remember

1. The factors *you* bring to therapy, such as your history, motivation and the support you have around you make the most difference and determine how likely therapy is to work.
2. In every field of human endeavour, effort counts. Therapy is no different.
3. Changing behaviour is difficult and often time consuming. Neuroscience tells us that the brain can change and, like the muscles in your body, it does so over time and in response to effort.
4. Motivation comes and goes. The key is to take action even when you don't feel like it. You're more likely to do that if you're clear about the purpose and values behind your actions.
5. Good therapy and a good therapist really help, but they can't do the work for you. For 167 hours of the week, you're on your own.
6. There are different phases of change. Sometimes you're getting ready to make change, or you're planning actions, and at other times you're maintaining gains. Therapy can help at every stage. Knowing where you are in the phases of change predicts success.
7. The six questions that make up the Readiness for Therapy questionnaire will help you assess how ready you are to begin therapy. No one is ever 100% ready. If you're really not ready, don't start; you'll be wasting your time and money. But if you are ready, do it.
8. Therapy is expensive, but therapy can cost the equivalent of a take-away coffee, croissant and a sandwich every working day for a week. Breakfast at home and take a packed lunch to work.
9. More than three-quarters of people benefit from therapy, and while outcomes can never be guaranteed, the odds are stacked in your favour if you're clear about what type of therapy and therapist will suit you and you're ready to change and willing to work hard.
10. For most people, most of the time, with most problems, therapy is well worth it.

Further reading and resources

This is a collection of resources we recommend to help you explore in more depth many of the subjects we've discussed in this book. This is by no means meant to be a comprehensive list – just a steer towards things we find helpful and interesting.

Mental health, personality and habits in general

Two brilliant books looking to further explore mental health are *Losing Our Minds: What mental health really is – and what it isn't*, by Lucy Foulkes (Bodley Head, 2021) and *Be Who You Want: Unlocking the science of personality change*, by Christian Jarrett (Robinson, 2021). Lucy Foulkes' book focuses on what mental health is and what it isn't. Christian Jarrett's book is about the science of personality and the scope of our ability to change who we are.

For habits and changing them, two great books are *How to Change: The science of getting from where you are to where you want to be*, by Katy Milkman (Vermilion, 2021) and *Good Habits, Bad Habits: The science of making positive changes that stick*, by Wendy Wood (Farrar, Straus & Giroux, 2019).

Diagnosis and understanding your specific problem

The main text used for diagnosing mental illness in the US is the *Diagnostic and Statistical Manual of Mental Disorders* (DSM) (American Psychiatric Association, 2013). You can buy the latest edition (DSM-5) at *www.appi.org/products/dsm*. But you're unlikely to want to, given its size and cost.

The World Health Organization's *International Classification of Diseases* (WHO, 2019) is used to diagnose mental health disorders across the globe, including in the UK. The latest edition (ICD-11) is available from here: *https://icd.who.int/en*. Section 6 focuses on mental health and is free to view on the website.

More user-friendly is the mental health charity Mind's website, which offers an excellent set of resources, including a simple explanation of a range of mental health problems: *www.mind.org.uk/information-support/types-of-mental-health-problems*

The Royal College of Psychiatrists website also offers a helpful section on its website: *www.rcpsych.ac.uk/mental-health/problems-disorders*

Different kinds of therapy

The NHS offers a useful set of resources about the different kinds of therapy, available at: *www.nhs.uk/mental-health/talking-therapies-medicine-treatments/talking-therapies-and-counselling/nhs-talking-therapies*

Mind's resources on the different types of therapy are also good: *www.mind.org.uk/information-support/drugs-and-treatments*

One of the best short introductions to cognitive behavioural therapy and how you can use it to help you is Seth Gillihan's *Cognitive Behavioural Therapy Made Simple* (Althea Press, 2018).

A good introduction to the emotional regulation skills techniques used in dialectical behavioural therapy is *Calming the Emotional Storm* by Sheri Van Dijk (New Harbinger Publications, 2012).

A good book on person-centred counselling, written for those considering training but also very helpful for those simply interested in knowing more about how it works, is *First Steps in Counselling*, by Pete Sanders, Paula J. Williams and Andy Rogers (PCCS Books, 2021, now in its fifth edition).

Any book by existential psychotherapist Irvin Yalom is highly recommended. His collections of case studies include *Staring into the Sun* (Piatkus, 2011) on mortality; *Love's Executioner* (Penguin, 2013) and *The Gift of Therapy* (Piatkus, 2010). All offer vivid glimpses into the workings of the human mind, heart and soul.

The Examined Life: How we lose and find ourselves (Vintage, 2014), by psychoanalyst Stephen Grosz, similarly captures insights into the human condition from its stories, only from a more psychoanalytic perspective.

Attachment and couples

If you're interested in exploring more about your attachment style, and what it means for your relationships, you can start with an online test, such as one from The Attachment Project, at: *www.attachmentproject.com*

Decent introductions to attachment theory are *Attached*, by Amir Levine and Rachel Heller (Tarcher Perigree, 2012) and, for couples, *Wired for Love*, by Stan Tankin (Echo Point Books, 2019). Another great book for couples looking to improve their relationship is *The Seven Principles for Making Marriage Work*, by John Gottman and Nan Silver (Orion Spring, 2018). *ACT with Love*, by Russ Harris (New Harbinger Publications, 2019), is another simple to read, jargon-free book that provides practical ways to improve your relationship – you can work through it on your own or with your partner.

Sue Gerhardt's *Why Love Matters* (Routledge, 2014, in its second revised edition) is a must for those interested in attachment, child development and how we can be set up for emotional breakdown by adverse child experiences.

Jacob Ham has produced a useful set of short videos on attachment theory, starting with secure attachment, which you can find on his YouTube channel: *www.youtube.com/watch?v=n2ypDPqs9A0*

Our own guide on 'How to understand and adapt your attachment style' is published on the *Psyche* digital magazine website, at: *https://psyche.co/guides/how-to-understand-and-adapt-your-attachment-style*

Anxiety

A brilliant first-hand account of what it's like to live with anxiety, and what helped, is Eleanor Morgan's *Anxiety for Beginners* (Pan Macmillan, 2017).

Depression

The best book we've read on depression is Andrew Solomon's *The Noonday Demon: An atlas of depression* (Scribner, 2015).

The journalist Oliver Kamm has written a great book called *Mending the Mind: The art and science of overcoming depression* (Orion Publishing, 2022) on overcoming his own clinical depression and how therapy helped him.

Addiction

Two books we'd recommend on addiction are *Out of the Wreck I Rise: A literary companion to recovery,* by Neil Steinberg and Sara Bader (University of Chicago Press, 2016), and *Unbroken Brain: A revolutionary new way of understanding addiction,* by Maia Szalavitz (Picador, 2017). Steinberg and Bader's book offers support and inspiration to anyone fighting addiction. Drawing on quotes from an array of literary figures, including Seneca, Shakespeare, Bukowski, Hemingway, Stephen King and Zadie Smith, and singers Billie Holiday and Bruce Springsteen, this lovely book sheds light on the notoriously difficult process of getting and staying sober. While the literary alcoholic is often romanticised, recovery from addiction is the true path of the hero. Szalavitz's book offers a new perspective on addiction, arguing that it's not a disease or a moral failing; rather that it's more like a developmental disorder, similar to autism or ADHD. The book explores her personal story of addiction alongside the science behind her views and the implications for treatment.

We wrote a piece on addiction on our website: *www.lcap.co.uk/articles/is-everything-you-know-about-addiction-really-wrong*

Trauma and post-traumatic resilience

We're fans of the 'Overcoming' series of books, which are part of the 'Reading Well, Books on Prescription' programme (*https://overcoming.co.uk/703/Reading-Well*), and supported by a range of professional bodies including Public Health England, NHS England and The Royal College of General Practitioners.

Overcoming Traumatic Stress, by Claudia Herbert (Robinson, 2017) is a practical self-help guide using CBT techniques.

Pete Walker's *Complex PTSD: From surviving to thriving* offers a practical deep dive into recovery from childhood neglect and abuse (Create Space, 2013).

George Bonanno has approached the subject from a different perspective, and his helpful book, *The End of Trauma,* focuses on how human resilience means most of us are surprisingly robust in the face of adversity (Basic Books, 2021).

Another classic text is Judith Herman's *Trauma and Recovery: The aftermath of violence – from domestic abuse to political terror* (Basic Books, 2015, first published 1992).

Obsessive compulsive disorder

A great self-help guide to help you understand and manage your own OCD is *Managing OCD with CBT for Dummies* by Katie d'Ath and Rob Wilson (For Dummies, 2016).

Psychiatric medication

One of the best overviews of the benefits and harms of psychiatric drugs is the companion book in this series, *A Straight Talking Introduction to Psychiatric Drugs: The truth about how they work and how to come off them*, by psychiatrist Joanna Moncrieff (PCCS Books, 2021).

The Royal College of Psychiatrists offers helpful resources on antidepressants and anti-anxiety medications on its website: *www.rcpsych.ac.uk/mental-health/treatments-and-wellbeing/antidepressants* and *www.rcpsych.ac.uk/mental-health/treatments-and-wellbeing/benzodiazepines*

Mind also has useful resources on psychiatric drugs on its website: *www.mind.org.uk/information-support/drugs-and-treatments*

Neurodiversity

If you're interested in getting a diagnosis of ADHD, you should speak to your GP in the first instance, but you can also take one of the number of online tests to see whether it's likely a formal assessment would be useful. This one from The ADHD Centre is a good start: *www.adhdcentre.co.uk/adhd-quiz*

Similarly, the clinical assessment of autism spectrum disorder (ASD) is lengthy, and should be conducted by someone with specialist training in that field. But there are several brief, initial screening tests available online, such as: *https://psychology-tools.com/test/raads-14*

Challenging the 'medical model' of mental health

A good introduction to the topic with regard to therapy is the edited work by Pete Sanders and Janet Tolan, *People Not Pathology: Freeing therapy from the medical model* (PCCS Books, 2023).

An energising critique of the medical model from the same publisher is *Drop the Disorder! Challenging the culture of psychiatric diagnosis*, edited by Jo Watson (PCCS Books, 2019).

Also in the same series as this book, *A Straight Talking Introduction to Psychiatric Diagnosis*, by Lucy Johnstone (PCCS Books, 2022, 2nd ed.), and *A Straight Talking Introduction to the Power Threat Meaning Framework*, by Mary Boyle and Lucy Johnstone (PCCS Books, 2020) together outline a less pathologising alternative to psychiatric diagnosis, pioneered by a group of radical psychologists.

Podcasts

The Gottman Institute has a really useful *Quick Tips About Relationships* bitesize podcast at: *www.gottman.com/podcast*

The *Dear Therapists* podcast offers a fly-on-the-wall experience of real therapy sessions: *https://lorigottlieb.com/podcast*

Nathan Filer is an author and mental health nurse. His podcast, *Why Do I Feel?*, combines theories and ideas about emotions with people's lived experiences: *www.nathanfiler.co.uk/why-do-i-feel*

Esther Perel's brilliant podcast *Where Shall We Begin?* offers you the opportunity to eavesdrop on real-life couples therapy: *www.estherperel.com/podcast*

Scott Barry Kaufman's *Psychology Podcast* is excellent. It's sometimes a little nerdy, but in a good way: *scottbarrykaufman.com/podcast*

References

Aggeler, M. (2019, July 9). Serena Williams started seeing a therapist after U.S. Open controversy. *The Cut*. https://www.thecut.com/2019/07/serena-williams-us-open-therapist.html

Aguirre, A. (2021, October 7). Adele on the other side. *Vogue*. https://www.vogue.com/article/adele-cover-november-2021

Albert, P.R. (2019). Adult neuroplasticity: A new 'cure' for major depression? *Journal of Psychiatry and Neuroscience, 44*(3), 147–150.

American Psychological Association. (2019, November 1). *What the evidence shows*. https://www.apa.org/monitor/2019/11/ce-corner-sidebar

American Psychological Association, Presidential Task Force on Evidence-Based Practice. (2006). Evidence-based practice in psychology. *American Psychologist, 61*(4), 271–285.

Ardito, R.B. & Rabellino, D. (2011). Therapeutic alliance and outcome of psychotherapy: Historical excursus, measurements, and prospects for research. *Frontiers in Psychology, 2*(270). https://doi.org/10.3389%2Ffpsyg.2011.00270

Arkowitz, H. & Lilienfeld, S.O. (2012, August 1). EMDR: Taking a closer look. *Scientific American*. https://www.scientificamerican.com/article/emdr-taking-a-closer-look

Baker, C. (2021). *Mental health statistics: prevalence, services and funding in England*. House of Commons Library, UK Parliament. https://commonslibrary.parliament.uk/research-briefings/sn06988

Baquet, D. (2017, November 29). Jay-Z & Dean Baquet: On therapy, politics, marriage, the state of rap and being a black man in America. *The New York Times Style Magazine*. https://www.nytimes.com/interactive/2017/11/29/t-magazine/jay-z-dean-baquet-interview.html

Barkham, M., Lutz, W. & Castonguay L.G. (Eds.). (2021b). *Bergin and Garfield's handbook of psychotherapy and behavior change* (7th ed.). Wiley.

Barkham, M., Saxon, D., Hardy, G.E., Bradburn, M., Galloway, D., Wickramasekera, N., Keetharuth, A.D., Bower, P., King, M., Elliott, R., Gabriel, L., Kellett, S., Shaw, S., Wilkinson, T., Connell, J., Harrison, P., Ardern, K., Bishop-Edwards, L., Ashley, K., Ohlse, S., Pilling, S., Waller, G. & Brazier, J.E. (2021a). Person-centred experiential therapy versus cognitive behavioural therapy delivered in the English Improving Access to Psychological Therapies service for the treatment of moderate or severe depression (PRaCTICED): A pragmatic, randomised, non-inferiority trial. *Lancet Psychiatry, 8*(6), 487–499.

Bartholomew, T.T., Joy, E.E. & Gundel, B.E. (2021). Clients' hope for counseling as a predictor of outcome in psychotherapy. *The Counseling Psychologist, 49*(8). https://doi.org/10.1177/00110000211033255

Batastini, A.B., Paprzycki, P., Jones, A.C.T. & MacLean N. (2020). Are videoconferenced mental and behavioral health services just as good as in-person? A meta-analysis of a fast-growing practice. *Clinical Psychology Review, 83,* 101944. https://doi.org/10.1016/j.cpr.2020.101944

Baumeister, R.F. & Tierney, J. (2012). *Willpower: Why self-control is the secret to success.* Penguin.

BBC News. (2021, March 15). *First ketamine-assisted psychotherapy Bristol clinic opens.* https://www.bbc.co.uk/news/uk-england-bristol-56170592

BBC News. (2022, November 29). *Quarter of 17-19-year-olds have probable mental disorder – study.* https://www.bbc.co.uk/news/health-63784751

Beck, J.S. (2005). *Cognitive therapy for challenging problems: What to do when the basics don't work.* Guilford Press.

Bellah, R.N., Madsen, R., Sullivan, W.M., Swidler, A. & Tipton, S.M. (2007). *Habits of the heart: Individualism and commitment in American life* (3rd ed.). University of California Press.

Benish, S.G., Imel, Z.E. & Wampold, B.E. (2008). The relative efficacy of bona fide psychotherapies for treating post-traumatic stress disorder: A meta-analysis of direct comparisons. *Clinical Psychology Review, 28*(5), 746–758.

Bogenschutz, M.P., Ross, S., Bhatt, S., Baron, T., Forcehimes, A.A., Laska, E., Mennenga, S.E., O'Donnell, K., Owens, L.T., Podrebarac, S., Rotrosen, J., Tonigan, J.T. & Worth, L. (2022). Percentage of heavy drinking days following psilocybin-assisted psychotherapy vs placebo in the treatment of adult patients with alcohol use disorder: A randomized clinical trial. *JAMA Psychiatry, 79*(10), 953–962.

Bonanno, G. (2021). *The end of trauma: How the new science of resilience is changing how we think about PTSD.* Basic Books.

Boswell, J.F., Sharpless, B.A., Greenberg, L.S., Heatherington, L., Huppert, J.D., Barber, J.P., Goldfried, M.R. & Castonguay, L.G. (2010). Schools of psychotherapy and the beginnings of a scientific approach.

In D.H. Barlow (Ed.), *The Oxford handbook of clinical psychology* (pp.98–127). Oxford University Press. https://doi.org/10.1093/oxfordhb/9780195366884.013.0006

Bradley, D. (2012, November 14). Why Gladwell's 10,000-hour rule is wrong. *BBC.* https://www.bbc.com/future/article/20121114-gladwells-10000-hour-rule-myth

Brewin, C.R. & Andrews, B. (2017, June 7). False memories of childhood abuse. *The Psychologist.* https://www.bps.org.uk/psychologist/false-memories-childhood-abuse

British Association for Counseling and Psychotherapy (BACP). (2019). *Public perceptions survey 2019.* https://www.bacp.co.uk/about-us/about-bacp/public-perception-survey-2019

British Association for Counselling and Psychotherapy (BACP). (2023, February 17). *2021-2022 workplace mapping survey.* https://www.bacp.co.uk/about-us/about-bacp/2021-2022-workplace-mapping-survey

Brookman-Byrne, A. (2022, March 28). The end of trauma as we know it? *The Psychologist.* https://www.bps.org.uk/psychologist/end-trauma-we-know-it

Carrard, I., Crépin, C., Rouget, P., Lam, T., Golay, A. & Van der Linden, M. (2011). Randomised controlled trial of a guided self-help treatment on the Internet for binge eating disorder. *Behaviour Research and Therapy, 49*(8), 482–491.

Cartwright, C., Gibson, K., Read, J., Cowan, O. & Dehar, T. (2016). Long-term antidepressant use: Patient perspectives of benefits and adverse effects. *Patient Preference and Adherence, 10*, 1401–1407.

Centers for Disease Control and Prevention. (2013). Suicide among adults aged 35-64 years – United States, 1999–2010. *Morbidity and Mortality Weekly Report, 62*(17), 321–342.

Chow, D.L., Miller, S.D., Seidel, J.A., Kane, R.T., Thornton, J.A. & Andrews, W.P. (2015). The role of deliberate practice in the development of highly effective psychotherapists. *Psychotherapy, 52*(3), 337–345.

Clay, R.A. (2010). More than one way to measure. *Monitor on Psychology, 41*(8), 52. https://www.apa.org/monitor/2010/09/trials

Clear, J. (2018). *Atomic habits.* Random House.

COMPASS Pathways. (2022, May 23). *Positive data from phase IIb study shows potential of COMP360 psilocybin therapy in treatment-resistant depression.* American Psychiatric Association, COMPASS News Archive. https://compasspathways.com/compass-pathways-presents-largest-ever-study-of-psilocybin-therapy-at-american-psychiatric-association-annual-meeting/#:~:text=Adverse%20events%3A%20In%20this%20study,scores%20in%20any%20treatment%20group

Cooper, M., Messow, C.-M., McConnachie, A., Freire, E., Elliott, R., Heard, D., Williams, C. & Morrison, J. (2017). Patient preference as a predictor of outcomes in a pilot trial of person-centred counselling versus low-intensity cognitive behavioural therapy for persistent sub-threshold and mild depression. *Counselling Psychology Quarterly, 31*(4). https://doi.org/10.1080/09515070.2017.1329708

Cooper, M. & Norcross, J.C. (2015). A brief, multidimensional measure of clients' therapy preferences: The Cooper-Norcross Inventory of Preferences (C-NIP). *International Journal of Clinical and Health Psychology, 16*(1). https://doi.org/10.1016/j.ijchp.2015.08.003

Cooper, M. & Norcross, J.C. (2019). Cooper-Norcross Inventory of Preferences (C-NIP) v1.1. [Online.] *Pluralistic Practice.* https://pluralisticpractice.com/wp-content/uploads/2019/06/C-NIP1.1-2019-04-04-with-guidelines.pdf

Cooper, M., Norcross J.C., Raymond-Barker, B. & Hogan T. (2019). Psychotherapy preferences of laypersons and mental health professionals: Whose therapy is it? *Psychotherapy, 56*(2), 205–216.

Craig, C., Hiskey S. & Spector A. (2020). Compassion focused therapy: A systematic review of its effectiveness and acceptability in clinical populations. *Expert Review of Neurotherapeutics, 20*(4), 385–400.

Craske, M.G., Roy-Byrne, P.P., Stein, M.B., Sullivan, G., Sherbourne, C. & Bystritsky, A. (2009). Treatment for anxiety disorders: Efficacy to effectiveness to implementation. *Behaviour Research and Therapy, 47*(11), 931–937.

Crawley, J. & Grant, J. (2007). *Couple therapy: The self in the relationship.* Palgrave.

Cribb, J., Karjalainen, H. & Waters, T. (2022, July 6). *Big rise in claims means disability benefits bill 70% higher than expected – and claimants on average waiting five months to receive.* Institute for Fiscal Studies. https://ifs.org.uk/news/big-rise-claims-means-disability-benefits-bill-70-higher-expected-and-claimants-average

Cuijpers, P., Berking, M., Andersson, G., Quigley, L., Kleiboer, A. & Dobson, K. S. (2013). A meta-analysis of cognitive-behavioural therapy for adult depression, alone and in comparison with other treatments. *The Canadian Journal of Psychiatry, 58*(7), 376–385.

Cuijpers, P., Noma, H., Karyotaki, E., Vinkers, C. H., Cipriani, A. & Furukawa, T.A. (2020). A network meta-analysis of the effects of psychotherapies, pharmacotherapies and their combination in the treatment of adult depression. *World Psychiatry, 19*(1), 92–107.

da Costa, S.C., Oesterle T., Rummans, T.A., Richelson, E. & Gold, M. (2022). Psychedelic drugs for psychiatric disorders. *Journal of the Neurological Sciences, 15*(440), 120332. doi: 10.1016/j.jns.2022.120332

David, D., Cotet, C., Matu, S., Mogoase, C. & Stefan, S. (2018). 50 years of rational-emotive and cognitive-behavioral therapy: A systematic review and meta-analysis. *Journal of Clinical Psychology, 74*(3), 304–318.

Davidson, P.R. & Lutz, A. (2008). Buddha's brain: Neuroplasticity and meditation. *IEEE Signal Process Mag, 25*(1), 176–184.

Davidson, P.R. & Parker, K.C.H. (2001). Eye movement desensitization and reprocessing (EMDR): A meta-analysis. *Journal of Consulting and Clinical Psychology, 69*(2), 305–316.

Deaton, A. & Cartwright, N. (2016). *Understanding and misunderstanding randomized controlled trials*. Durham University Press.

de Shazer, S. (1985). *Keys to solution in brief therapy*. W.W. Norton & Co.

Devilly, G.J. & Borkovec, T.D. (2000). Psychometric properties of the Credibility/Expectancy Questionnaire. *Journal of Behavior Therapy and Experimental Psychiatry, 31*(2), 73–86.

Dimidjian S. (Ed.). (2019). *Evidence-based practice in action: Bridging clinical science and intervention*. Guilford Press.

Dinneen, J. (2020, July 8). I chatted with a therapy bot to ease my covid fears. It was bizarre. *OneZero*. https://onezero.medium.com/i-chatted-with-a-therapy-bot-to-ease-my-covid-fears-it-was-bizarre-ccd908264660

Dryden, W. (2019). *Single-session therapy: Distinctive features*. Routledge.

Duckworth A.L, Peterson, C., Matthews, M.D. & Kelly, D.R. (2007). Grit: Perseverance and passion for long-term goals. *Journal of Personality and Social Psychology, 92*(6), 1087–1101.

Dweck, C. (2018, June 26). Growth mindset interventions yield impressive results. *The Conversation*. https://theconversation.com/growth-mindset-interventions-yield-impressive-results-97423

Eastal, S. (Dir.). (2021). *The psychedelic drug trial*. [TV series]. BBC. https://www.bbc.co.uk/programmes/m000w7bq

Ehlers, A., Bisson, J., Clark, D.M., Creamer, M., Pilling, S., Richards, D., Schnurr, P.P., Turner, S. & Yulea, W. (2010). Do all psychological treatments really work the same in posttraumatic stress disorder? *Clinical Psychology Review, 30*(2), 269–276.

Eisler, I., Dare, C., Hodes, M., Russell, G., Dodge, E. & Le Grange, D. (2000). Family therapy for adolescent anorexia nervosa: The results of a controlled comparison of two family interventions. *Journal of Child Psychology and Psychiatry, 41*(6), 727–736.

Elkins, D.N. (2009). The medical model in psychotherapy: Its limitations and failures. *Journal of Humanistic Psychology, 49*(1), 66–84.

Elliott, R., Bohart, A.C., Watson, J.C. & Murphy, D. (2018). Therapist empathy and client outcome: An updated meta-analysis. *Psychotherapy, 55*(4), 399–410.

Emmelkamp, P.M.G. & Meyerbröker, K. (2021). Virtual reality therapy in mental health. *Annual Review of Clinical Psychology, 17*, 495–519.

Erekson, D.M., Clayson, R., Park, S.Y. & Tass, S. (2020). Therapist effects on early change in psychotherapy in a naturalistic setting. *Psychotherapy Research, 30*(1), 68–78.

Ericsson, A. & Pool, R. (2016, April 10). Malcolm Gladwell got us wrong: Our research was key to the 10,000-hour rule, but here's what got oversimplified. *Salon.* https://www.salon.com/2016/04/10/malcolm_gladwell_got_us_wrong_our_research_was_key_to_the_10000_hour_rule_but_heres_what_got_oversimplified/

Ericsson, K.A., Prietula, M.J. & Cokely, E.T. (2007, July-August). The making of an expert. *Harvard Business Review.* https://hbr.org/2007/07/the-making-of-an-expert

Ernest, P., Jandrain, B. & Scheen, A.J. (2015). Strengths and weaknesses of randomised control trials: Evolving changes according to personalised medicine. *Revue Médicale de Liège, 70*(5–6), 232–236.

Euba, R. (2019, July 19). Humans aren't designed to be happy – so stop trying. *The Conversation.* https://theconversation.com/humans-arent-designed-to-be-happy-so-stop-trying-119262

Eubanks, C.F. & Goldfried, M.R. (2019). A principle-based approach to psychotherapy integration. In J.C. Norcross & M.R. Goldfried (Eds.), *Handbook of Psychotherapy Integration* (3rd ed.) (pp.88–108). Oxford University Press.

Eyal, N. (2016, November 23). Have we been thinking about willpower the wrong way for 30 years? *Harvard Business Review.* https://hbr.org/2016/11/have-we-been-thinking-about-willpower-the-wrong-way-for-30-years

Farber, B., Suzuki, J. & Lynch, D.A. (2018). Positive regard and psychotherapy outcome: A meta-analytic review. *Psychotherapy Theory Research Practice Training, 55*(4), 411–423.

Filer, N. (2019). *This book will change your mind about mental health.* Faber.

Firth, J., Marx, W., Dash, S., Carney, R., Teasdale, S.B., Solmi, M., Stubbs, B., Schuch, F.B., Carvalho, A. F., Jacka, F. & Sarris, J. (2019). The effects of dietary improvement on symptoms of depression and anxiety: A meta-analysis of randomized controlled trials. *Psychosomatic Medicine, 81*(3), 265–280.

Fischer, M. (2021, March 29). The therapy-app fantasy: An overwhelming demand for counseling has spawned slickly marketed companies promising a service they cannot possibly provide. *The Cut.* https://www.thecut.com/article/mental-health-therapy-apps.html

Fisher B., Wolmark N., Redmond C., Deutsch M. & Fisher E.R. (1981). Findings from NSABP protocol no. b-04: Comparison of radical mastectomy with alternative treatments. II. The clinical and biologic significance of medial-central breast cancers. *Cancer, 48*(8), 1863–1872.

Fonagy, P., Lemma, A., Target, M., O'Keeffe S., Constantinou M.P., Wurman, T.V., Luyten, P., Allison, E., Roth, A., Cape, J. & Pilling, S. (2020). Dynamic interpersonal therapy for moderate to severe depression: A pilot randomized controlled and feasibility trial. *Psychological Medicine, 50*(6), 1010–1019.

Foulkes, L. (2021). *Losing our minds: What mental illness really is – and what it isn't.* Bodley Head.

Fraley, R.C. (2016). Attachment stability from infancy to adulthood: Meta-analysis and dynamic modeling of developmental mechanisms. *Personality and Social Psychology Review, 6*(2). https://doi.org/10.1207/S15327957PSPR0602_03

Frances, A. (2013). *Saving normal: An insider's revolt against out-of-control psychiatric diagnosis, DSM-5, Big Pharma, and the medicalization of ordinary life.* William Morrow & Co.

Fulwiler, M. (2012, July 2). Managing conflict: Solvable vs. perpetual problems. *The Gottman Institute.* https://www.gottman.com/blog/managing-conflict-solvable-vs-perpetual-problems/

Geller, L.W. (2014, August 8). Katherine Milkman on why fresh starts matter. *strategy+business.* https://www.strategy-business.com/article/00266

Ghomi, M., Wrightman, M., Ghaemian, A., Grey, N., Pickup, T. & Richardson, T. (2020). Development and validation of the Readiness for Therapy Questionnaire (RTQ). *Behavioural and Cognitive Psychotherapy, 49*(4), 413–425.

Gilbert, P. (2009, May 3). Moving beyond cognitive behaviour therapy. *The Psychologist.* https://www.bps.org.uk/psychologist/moving-beyond-cognitive-behaviour-therapy

Gilbody, S., Littlewood, E., Hewitt, C., Brierley, G., Tharmanathan, P., Araya, R., Barkham, M., Bower, P., Cooper, C., Gask, L., Kessler, D., Lester, H., Lovell, K., Parry, G., Richards, D. A., Andersen, P., Brabyn, S., Knowles, S., Shepherd, C., Tallon, D., White, D. & REEACT Team. (2015). Computerised cognitive behaviour therapy (cCBT) as treatment for depression in primary care (REEACT trial): Large scale pragmatic randomised controlled trial. *British Medical Journal, 351*, 1–13.

Gingerich, W.J. & Peterson, L.T. (2013). Effectiveness of solution-focused brief therapy: A systematic qualitative review of controlled outcome studies. *Research on Social Work Practice, 23*(3). https://doi.org/10.1177/1049731512470859

Goldberg, S.B., Lam, S.U., Simonsson, O., Torous, J. & Sun, S. (2022). Mobile phone-based interventions for mental health: A systematic meta-review of 14 meta-analyses of randomized controlled trials. *PLOS Digital Health.* https://doi.org/10.1371/journal.pdig.0000002

Goldstein, J. (2019, April 3). Justin Bieber shares photo from therapy session: 'It's cool to have a healthy mind and emotions'. *People.com.* https://people.com/music/justin-bieber-attends-therapy-session-cool-healthy-mind/

Gottman, J.M. (2007). *Why marriages succeed or fail.* Bloomsbury Publishing.

Greene, A. (2012, July 23). Bruce Springsteen battled depression, suicidal thoughts in early 1980s. *Rolling Stone.* https://www.rollingstone.com/music/music-news/bruce-springsteen-battled-depression-suicidal-thoughts-in-early-1980s-64354

Halford, B. (2022, March 6). Drug companies are investing big in psychedelics, but can they engineer out the trip? *c&en.* https://cen.acs.org/pharmaceuticals/drug-development/Drug-companies-investing-big-psychedelics/100/i9#:~:text=The%20drug%20industry%20is%20tuning,mushroom%20in%20the%20coming%20years

Hallas, D., Spratling, R. & Fletcher, J. (2021). Methodological analysis: Randomized controlled trials for Pfizer and Moderna COVID-19 vaccines. *Journal of Pediatric Health Care, 35*(4), 443–448.

Harandi, T.F., Taghinasab, M.M. & Nayeri, T.D. (2017). The correlation of social support with mental health: A meta-analysis. *Electron Physician, 9*(9), 5212–5222.

Hariton, E. & Locascio, J.L. (2018). Randomised controlled trials – the gold standard for effectiveness research. *BJOG, 125*(13), 1716.

Harris-Fry, N. (2017, March 28). Here's how close your gym needs to be to ensure you go regularly. *Coach Web.* www.coachweb.com/fitness/6456/here-s-how-close-your-gym-needs-to-be-to-ensure-you-go-regularly

Haynes, L., Service, O., Goldacre, B. & Torgerson, D. (2012). *Test, learn, adapt: Developing public policy with randomised controlled trials.* Behavioural Insights Team, Cabinet Office. https://assets.publishing.service.gov.uk/government/uploads/system/uploads/attachment_data/file/62529/TLA-1906126.pdf

Health and Safety Executive (HSE). (2022). *Working days lost in Great Britain.* HSE. https://www.hse.gov.uk/statistics/dayslost.htm

Hiatt, B. & Nodland, N. (2019, March 26). Growing up 'Game of Thrones'. *Rolling Stone.* https://www.rollingstone.com/tv-movies/tv-movie-features/game-of-thrones-cover-story-maisie-williams-sophie-turner-812203

Hill, C.E., Knox, S. & Pinto-Coelho, K.G. (2018). Therapist self-disclosure and immediacy: A qualitative meta-analysis. *Psychotherapy, 55*(4), 445–460.

Iacobucci, G. (2019). NHS prescribed record number of antidepressants last year. *British Medical Journal, 364*, l1508. https://doi.org/10.1136/bmj.l1508

Imel, Z.E. & Wampold, B.E. (2008). The importance of treatment and the science of common factors in psychotherapy. In S.D. Brown & R.W. Lent (Eds.), *Handbook of counseling psychology* (pp.249–266). John Wiley & Sons.

Institute for Quality and Efficiency in Health Care. (2020, June 18). Depression: How effective are antidepressants? *InformedHealth.org*. https://www.ncbi.nlm.nih.gov/books/NBK361016

Irvine, A., Drew, P., Bower, P., Brooks, H., Gellatly, J., Armitage, C.J., Barkham, M., McMillan, D. & Beed, P. (2020). Are there interactional differences between telephone and face-to-face psychological therapy? A systematic review of comparative studies. *Journal of Affective Disorders, 265*, 120–131.

Jackson, C. (2023). The big issue: Is working with psychedelics the future of therapy? *Therapy Today, 34*(6), 18–22.

Jarrett, C. (2021). *Be who you want: Unlocking the science of personality change*. Robinson.

Johnstone, L. (2021). *A straight talking introduction to psychiatric diagnosis* (Rev. 2nd ed.). PCCS Books.

Johnstone, L. & Boyle, M., with Cromby, J., Dillon, J., Harper, D., Kinderman, P., Longden, E., Pilgrim, D., & Read, J. (2018). *The Power Threat Meaning Framework: Towards the identification of patterns in emotional distress, unusual experiences and troubled or troubling behaviour, as an alternative to functional psychiatric diagnosis*. British Psychological Society. www.bps.org.uk/power-threat-meaning-framework

Kabat-Zinn, J. (2013). *Full catastrophe living*. Bantam.

Kamenetz, A. (2016, May 25). MacArthur 'genius' Angela Duckworth responds to a new critique of grit. *nprED*. https://www.npr.org/sections/ed/2016/05/25/479172868/angela-duckworth-responds-to-a-new-critique-of-grit

Kazantzis, N., Luong, H.K., Usatoff, A.S., Impala, T., Yew, R.Y. & Hofmann, S.G. (2018). The processes of cognitive behavioral therapy: A review of meta-analyses. *Cognitive Therapy and Research, 42*(5).

Kerner, I. (2021). *So tell me about the last time you had sex*. Scribe.

Kertz, S.J., Kelly, J.M., Stevens, K.T., Schrock, M. & Danitz, S.B. (2017). A review of free iPhone applications designed to target anxiety and worry. *Journal of Technology in Behavioral Science, 2*, 61–70.

Kolden, G.G., Wang C., Austin, S.B., Chang, Y. & Klein, M.H. (2018). Congruence/genuineness: A meta-analysis. *Psychotherapy, 55*(4), 424–433.

Kortlever, J.T.P., Ottenhoff, J.S.E., Vagner, G.A., Ring, D. & Reichel, L.M. (2019). Visit duration does not correlate with perceived physician empathy. *The Journal of Bone and Joint Surgery, 101*(4), 296–301.

Kraus, D.R., Bentley, J.H., Alexander, P.C., Boswell, J. F., Constantino, M.J., Baxter, E.E. & Castonguay, L.G. (2016). Predicting therapist effectiveness from their own practice-based evidence. *Journal of Consulting and Clinical Psychology, 84*(6), 473–483.

Kumar, V., Sattar, Y., Bseiso, A., Khan, S. & Rutkofsky, I.H. (2017). The effectiveness of internet-based cognitive behavioral therapy in treatment of psychiatric disorders. *Cureus, 9*(8). https://pubmed.ncbi.nlm.nih.gov/29098136/

Kuyken, W., Ball, S., Crane, C., Ganguli, P., Jones, B., Montero-Marin, J., Nuthall, E., Raja, A., Taylor, L., Tudor, K., Viner, R.M., Allwood, M., Aukland, L., Dunning, D., Casey, T., Dalrymple, N., De Wilde, K., Farley, E., Harper, J. et al. (2022). Effectiveness of universal school-based mindfulness training compared with normal school provision on teacher mental health and school climate: Results of the MYRIAD cluster randomised controlled trial. *Child and Adolescent Mental Health, 25*, 125–134.

Lambert, M.J. (2013). The efficacy and effectiveness of psychotherapy. In M.J. Lambert (Ed.), *Bergin and Garfield's handbook of psychotherapy and behaviour change* (6th ed.) (pp.169–218). Wiley.

Layard, R. (2005, January 20). *Mental health: Britain's biggest social problem?* Paper presented at the No.10 Strategy Unit Seminar on Mental Health. http://eprints.lse.ac.uk/47428

Layard, R. & Clark, D.M. (2015a). *Thrive: The power of psychological therapy.* Penguin.

Layard, R., & Clark, D.M. (2015b). Why more psychological therapy would cost nothing. *Frontiers in Psychology, 6*, 1713.

Lebow, J. & Snyder, D.K. (2022). Couple therapy in the 2020s: Current status and emerging developments. *Family Process, 61*(4), 1359–1385.

Lemma, A., Target, M. & Fonagy, P. (2011). *Brief dynamic interpersonal therapy: A clinician's guide*. Oxford Academic Press.

Lilienfeld, S.O. & Arkowitz, H. (2012, September 1). Are all psychotherapies created equal? *Scientific American.* https://www.scientificamerican.com/article/are-all-psychotherapies-created-equal/

Lilienfeld, S.O., McKay, S. & Hollon, S.D. (2018). Why randomised controlled trials of psychological treatments are still essential. *The Lancet, 5*(7), 536–538.

Lim, G.Y., Tam, W.W., Lu, Y., Ho, C.S., Zhang, M.W. & Ho, R.C. (2018). Prevalence of depression in the community from 30 countries between 1994 and 2014. *Scientific Reports, 8*(1), 2861.

Linden, D. (2006). How psychotherapy changes the brain – the contribution of functional neuroimaging. *Molecular Psychiatry, 11*, 528–538.

Linehan, M.M., Dimeff, L.A., Reynolds, S.K., Comtois, K.A., Welch, S.S., Heagerty, P. & Kivlahan, D.R. (2002). Dialectical behavior therapy versus comprehensive validation therapy plus 12-step for the treatment of opioid dependent women meeting criteria for borderline personality disorder. *Drug and Alcohol Dependence, 67*(1), 13–26.

Locke, E.A., Shaw, K.N., Saari, L.M. & Latham, G.P. (1981). Goal setting and task performance: 1969–1980. *Psychological Bulletin, 90*(1), 125–152.

London Centre for Applied Psychology. (2022). *Clients tell us they want more challenge. Why do therapists avoid it?* https://www.lcap.co.uk/articles/clients-tell-us-they-want-more-challenge-why-do-therapists-avoid-it

Luborsky, L, Rosenthal, R, Diguer, L. & Andrusyna, T.P. (2002). The Dodo bird verdict is alive and well – mostly. *Clinical Psychology Science and Practice, 9*(1), 2–12.

Luo, C., Sanger, N., Singhal, N., Pattrick, K., Shams, I., Shahid, H., Hoang, P., Schmidt, J., Lee, J., Haber, S., Puckering, M., Buchanan, N., Lee, P., Ng, K., Sun, S., Kheyson, S., Cho-Yan Chung, D., Sanger, S., Thabane, L. & Samaang, Z. (2020). A comparison of electronically-delivered and face to face cognitive behavioural therapies in depressive disorders: A systematic review and meta-analysis. *EClinicalMedicine, 24,* 100442. https://doi.org/10.1016/j.eclinm.2020.100442

Manby, C. (2018, August 29). What is it that you're really afraid of? *The Independent.* https://www.independent.co.uk/life-style/fear-spiders-heights-snakes-buttons-phobia-arachnid-arachnophobia-a8495776.html

Marcelle, E.T., Nolting, L., Hinshaw, S.P. & Aguilera, A. (2019). Effectiveness of a multimodal digital psychotherapy platform for adult depression: A naturalistic feasibility study. *JMIR MHealth and UHealth, 7*(1). https://doi.org/10.2196/10948

Mayou, R.A., Ehlers, A. & Hobbs, M. (2000). Psychological debriefing for road traffic accident victims. Three-year follow-up of a randomised controlled trial. *British Journal of Psychiatry, 176*, 589–593.

McQuaid, A., Sanatinia, R., Farquharson, L., Shah, P., Quark, A., Baldwin, D.S. & Crawford, M. (2021). Patient experience of lasting negative effects of psychological interventions for anxiety and depression in secondary mental health care services: A national cross-sectional study. *BMC Psychiatry, 21*(578). https://doi.org/10.1186/s12888-021-03588-2

Milkman, K. (2021). *How to change: The science of getting from where you are to where you want to be.* Vermillion.

Millea, H. (2015, August 11). 4 things we learned about Keira Knightley that made us fall in love with her. *Elle*. https://www.elle.com/fashion/a29679/keira-knightley-elle-2015

Miller, W.R. & Moyers, T.B. (2021). *Effective psychotherapists: Clinical skills that improve client outcomes*. Guilford Press.

Miller, W.R. & Rose, G.S. (2009). Toward a theory of motivational interviewing. *American Psychologist, 64*(6), 527–537.

Miller, W.R. & Tonigan, J.S. (1997). Assessing drinkers' motivation for change: The Stages of Change Readiness and Treatment Eagerness Scale (SOCRATES). In G.A. Marlatt & G.R. VandenBos (Eds.), *Addictive behaviors: Readings on etiology, prevention, and treatment* (pp.355–369). American Psychological Association.

Mind. (2018, June 5). *40 per cent of all GP appointments about mental health.* [Online.] Mind. www.mind.org.uk/news-campaigns/news/40-per-cent-of-all-gp-appointments-about-mental-health/

Mind. (2020, June). *Mental health facts and statistics.* [Online.] Mind. https://www.mind.org.uk/information-support/types-of-mental-health-problems/statistics-and-facts-about-mental-health/how-common-are-mental-health-problems/

Moncrieff, J., Cooper, R.E., Stockmann, T., Amendola, S., Hengartner M.P. & Horowitz, M.A. (2022). The serotonin theory of depression: A systematic umbrella review of the evidence. *Molecular Psychiatry.* https://doi.org/10.1038/s41380-022-01661-0

Moncrieff, J. & Timimi, S. (2013). The social and cultural construction of psychiatric knowledge: an analysis of NICE guidelines on depression and ADHD. *Anthropology & Medicine, 20*(1), 59–71.

Moyers, T.B. & Miller, W.R. (2012). Is low therapist empathy toxic? *Psychology of Addictive Behaviors, 27*(3), 878–884.

Mumford, G. (2015). *The mindful athlete: Secrets to pure performance.* Parallax Press.

National Institute for Health and Care Excellence. (NICE). (2011). *Generalised anxiety disorder and panic disorder in adults: management.* NICE. www.nice.org.uk/guidance/cg113/chapter/Recommendations

National Institute for Health and Care Excellence. (NICE). (2017). *Eating disorders: recognition and treatment.* NICE. www.nice.org.uk/guidance/ng69/chapter/recommendations

National Institute for Health and Care Excellence. (NICE). (2018). *Post-traumatic stress disorder.* (NG116). NICE. www.nice.org.uk/guidance/ng116/chapter/recommendations

National Institute for Health and Care Excellence (NICE). (2022). *Depression in adults: Treatment and management.* www.nice.org.uk/guidance/ng222/chapter/Recommendations

National Institute for Health and Care Excellence (NICE). (2023). *Digitally enabled therapies for adults with depression: Early value assessment.* NICE. www.nice.org.uk/guidance/hte8

Navasky, V.S. & Cerf, C. (1998). *The experts speak: The definitive compendium of authoritative misinformation.* Random House.

Nechamkin, S. (2018, November 12). Michelle Obama says she and Barack went to couples therapy. *The Cut.* https://www.thecut.com/2018/11/michelle-obama-says-she-and-barack-went-to-couples-therapy.html

New Zealand Government. (2016). *Scared straight: Evidence brief.* New Zealand Government. https://www.justice.govt.nz/assets/Scared-Straight.pdf

NHS. (2022a, February 11). *Self-help therapies.* [Online.] https://www.nhs.uk/mental-health/talking-therapies-medicine-treatments/talking-therapies-and-counselling/self-help-therapies/

NHS. (2022b, February 17). *Types of talking therapy.* [Online.] https://www.nhs.uk/mental-health/talking-therapies-medicine-treatments/talking-therapies-and-counselling/types-of-talking-therapies/

NHS Business Services Authority. (2022, July 7). *Medicines used in mental health – England – Quarterly summary statistics January to March 2022.* [Online.]https://www.nhsbsa.nhs.uk/statistical-collections/medicines-used-mental-health-england/medicines-used-mental-health-england-quarterly-summary-statistics-january-march-2022

NHS Digital. (2021, November, 21). *New statistics released on talking therapies in England.* [Online.] https://digital.nhs.uk/news/2021/new-statistics-released-on-talking-therapies-in-england

NHS Digital. (2022a). *Mental health bulletin, 2021–22 Annual report.* [Online.] https://digital.nhs.uk/data-and-information/publications/statistical/mental-health-bulletin/2021-22-annual-report

NHS Digital. (2022b). *Psychological therapies, Annual report on the use of IAPT services, 2021-22.* https://digital.nhs.uk/data-and-information/publications/statistical/psychological-therapies-annual-reports-on-the-use-of-iapt-services/annual-report-2021-22

Nikkhah, R. (2010, March 28). Emma Thompson says work saved her from 'going under' in her battle with depression. *The Telegraph.* https://www.telegraph.co.uk/news/celebritynews/7530122/Emma-Thompson-says-work-saved-her-from-going-under-in-her-battle-with-depression.html

Norcross, J.C. (2012). *Changeology: 5 steps to realizing your goals and resolutions.* Simon & Schuster.

Norcross, J.C. & Goldfried, M.R. (2019). *Handbook of psychotherapy integration* (3rd ed.). Oxford University Press.

Norcross, J.C. & Lambert, M.J. (2019). Evidence-based psychotherapy relationships: The third task force. In J.C. Norcross & M.J. Lambert (Eds.), *Psychotherapy relationships that work: Evidence-based therapist contributions* (pp. 1–23). Oxford University Press.

Norcross, J.C. & Wampold, B.E. (2018). A new therapy for each patient: Evidence-based relationships and responsiveness. *Journal of Clinical Psychology, 74*(11), 1889–1906.

Nutt, D. (2019). Psychedelic drugs – a new era in psychiatry? *Dialogues in Clinical Neuroscience, 21*(2), 139–147. doi: 10.31887/DCNS.2019.21.2/dnutt

Nutt, D., Erritzoe, D. & Carhart-Harris, R. (2020). Psychedelic psychiatry's brave new world. *Cell, 181*(1), 24–28.

O'Keefe, P.A., Dweck, C. & Walton, G. (2018, September 10). Having a growth mindset makes it easier to develop new interests. *Harvard Business Review.* https://hbr.org/2018/09/having-a-growth-mindset-makes-it-easier-to-develop-new-interests

Okiishi, J., Lambert, M.J., Nielsen, S.L. & Ogles, B.M. (2003). Waiting for supershrink: An empirical analysis of therapist effects. *Clinical Psychology & Psychotherapy, 10*(6), 361–373.

Organisation for Economic Co-operation and Development. (2021, June 8). *Improving mental health care key to COVID-19 pandemic recovery.* [Online.] https://www.oecd.org/health/improving-mental-health-care-key-to-covid-19-pandemic-recovery.htm

Owen, J., Drinane, J.M., Kivlighan, M., Miller, S.D., Kopta, M. & Imel, Z. (2019). Are high-performing therapists both effective and consistent? A test of therapist expertise. *Journal of Consulting and Clinical Psychology, 87*(12), https://doi.org/10.1037/ccp0000437

Owens, M.T. & Tanner, K.D. (2017). Teaching as brain changing: Exploring connections between neuroscience and innovative teaching. *CBE–Life Sciences Education, 16*(2). https://doi.org/10.1187/cbe.17-01-0005

Pachankis, J. E., & Goldfried, M.R. (2007). An integrative, principle-based approach to psychotherapy. In S. Hofmann & J. Weinberger (Eds.), *The Art and Science of Psychotherapy* (pp.49–68). Routledge.

Patten, S.B., Williams, J.V.A., Lavorato, D.H., Modgill, G., Jetté N. & Eliasziw, M. (2008). Major depression as a risk factor for chronic disease incidence: longitudinal analyses in a general population cohort. *General Hospital Psychiatry*, *30*(5), 407–413.

Powers, M.B. & Emmelkamp, P.M.G. (2008). Virtual reality exposure therapy for anxiety disorders: A meta-analysis. *Journal of Anxiety Disorders, 22*(3), 561–569.

Pritchett, D., Sontheimer, H., Shivers, B., Dolan B., Ymer, S., Kettenmann, H., Schofield, P.R. & Seeburg, P.H. (1989). Importance of a novel GABAA receptor subunit for benzodiazepine pharmacology. *Nature, 338*, 582–585.

Prochaska, J.O. & DiClemente, C.C. (1986). Toward a comprehensive model of change. In W.R. Miller & N. Heather (Eds.), *Treating addictive behaviors: Processes of change* (pp.3–27). Plenum Press.

Project MATCH (1993). Project MATCH (Matching Alcoholism Treatment to Client Heterogeneity): Rationale and methods for a multisite clinical trial matching patients to alcoholism treatment. *Alcohol: Clinical and Experimental Research, (17)*6, 1130–1145.

Purser, R.E. (2019). *McMindfulness: How mindfulness became the new capitalist spirituality*. Repeater Books.

Putnam, R.D. (1995). Bowling alone: America's declining social capital. *Journal of Democracy*, *6*(1), 65–78.

Ramirez, I. (1990). Why do sugars taste good? *Neuroscience & Biobehavioural Reviews, 14*(2), 125–134.

Redelmeier, D.A., Ferris, L.E., Tu, J.V., Hux, J.E. & Schull M.J. (2001). Problems for clinical judgement: Introducing cognitive psychology as one more basic science. *CMAJ, 164*(3), 358–360.

Ridgway, N., & Williams, C. (2011). Cognitive behavioural therapy self-help for depression: An overview. *Journal of Mental Health, 20*(6). https://doi.org /10.3109/09638237.2011.613956.

Ritchie, S. (2022, April 14). Everything you need to know about psychedelics and mental illness. *Science Fictions*. https://www.sciencefictions.org/p/psychedelics

Rollnick, S., Miller, W.R. & Butler, C. C. (2009). Motivational interviewing in health care: Helping patients change behavior. *American Journal of Pharmaceutical Education, 73*(7), 127.

Royal College of Psychiatrists. (2021a, December). *Our workforce census*. [Online.]https://www.rcpsych.ac.uk/improving-care/workforce/our-workforce-census

Royal College of Psychiatrists. (2021b, November). *Coping after a traumatic event*. [Online.] https://www.rcpsych.ac.uk/mental-health/problems-disorders/coping-after-a-traumatic-event

Royal College of Psychiatrists. (2022, October 10). *Hidden waits force more than three quarters of mental health patients to seek help from emergency services*. [Online.] www.rcpsych.ac.uk/news-and-features/latest-news/detail/2022/10/10/hidden-waits-force-more-than-three-quarters-of-mental-health-patients-to-seek-help-from-emergency-services

Salkovskis, P. (2001). Review: Eye movement desensitisation and reprocessing is not better than exposure therapies for anxiety or trauma. *Journal of Consulting and Clinical Psychology, 69*, 305–316.

Sanders, P. & Tolan, J. (Eds.). (2023). *People not pathology: Freeing therapy from the medical model.* PCCS Books.

Sanders, P., Williams, P.J. & Rogers, A. (2021). *First steps in counselling: An introductory companion* (5th ed.). PCCS Books.

Sareen, J. (2014). Posttraumatic stress disorder in adults: Impact, comorbidity, risk factors, and treatment. *Canadian Journal of Psychiatry, 59*(9), 460–467.

Schizofrenidagene. (2016, November 17). *Psychotherapy debate with Peter Fonagy and Bruce Wampold at the Nordic Conference on Mental Health.* [Video]. YouTube. www.youtube.com/watch?app=desktop&v=U5fhhAZnduU

Scott A.J., Webb T.L., Martyn-St James, M., Rowse, G. & Weich S. (2021). Improving sleep quality leads to better mental health: A meta-analysis of randomised controlled trials. *Sleep Medicine Reviews, 60*, 101556.

Seligman, M.E.P. (1995). The effectiveness of psychotherapy. *American Psychologist, 50*(12), 965–974.

Shedler, J. (2017, November 19). Selling bad therapy to trauma victims. *Psychology Today*. https://www.psychologytoday.com/gb/blog/psychologically-minded/201711/selling-bad-therapy-trauma-victims

Shedler, J. (2018). Where is the evidence for 'evidence-based' therapy? *Psychiatric Clinics of North America, 41*, 319–329.

Sherwood, H. & Giuffrida, A. (2017, September 1). Pope reveals he had weekly psychoanalysis sessions at age 42. *The Guardian*. www.theguardian.com/world/2017/sep/01/pope-francis-psychoanalysis

Skapinakis, P., Caldwell, D., Hollingworth, W., Bryden, P., Fineberg, N., Salkovskis, P., Welton, N., Baxter, H., Kessler, D., Churchill R., & Lewis, G. (2016). A systematic review of the clinical effectiveness and cost-effectiveness of pharmacological and psychological interventions for the management of obsessive compulsive disorder in children/adolescents and adults. *Health Technology Assessment, 20*(43). https://doi.org/10.3310/hta20430

Spanos, B. (2022, August 22). How Harry Styles became the world's most wanted man. *Rolling Stone*. https://www.rollingstone.com/music/music-features/harry-styles-harrys-house-dont-worry-darling-my-policeman-cover-1397290/

Spencer, J., Goode, J., Penix, E.A., Trusty, W. & Swift, J.K. (2019). Developing a collaborative relationship with clients during the initial sessions of psychotherapy. *Psychotherapy, 56*(1), 7–10.

Strawn, J.R., Geracioti, L., Rajdev, N., Clemenza, K. & Levine, A. (2018). Pharmacotherapy for generalized anxiety disorder in adults and pediatric patients: An evidence-based treatment review. *Expert Opinion on Pharmacotherapy, 19*(10), 1057–1070.

Sucala, M., Cuijpers, P., Muench, F., Cardoş, R., Soflau, R., Dobrean, A., Achimas-Cadariu, P. & David, D. (2017). Anxiety: There is an app for that. A systematic review of anxiety apps. *Depression & Anxiety, 34*(6), 518–525.

Svenson, O. (1981). Are we all less risky and more skillful than our fellow drivers? *Acta Psychologica, (47)*2, 143–148.

Swift, J.K. & Callahan, J.L. (2009a). The impact of client treatment preferences on outcome: a meta-analysis. *Journal of Clinical Psychology, 65*(4), 368–381.

Swift, J.K. & Callahan, J.L. (2009b). Early psychotherapy processes: An examination of client and trainee clinician perspective convergence. *Clinical Psychology & Psychotherapy, 16*(3), 228–236.

Swift, J.K., Callahan, J.L., Cooper, M. & Parkin, S. (2018). The impact of accommodating client preference in psychotherapy: A meta-analysis. *Journal of Clinical Psychology, 74*(1), 1924–1937. https://doi.org/10.1002/jclp.22680

Szasz, T. (1961). *The myth of mental illness: Foundations of a theory of personal conduct.* Harper & Row.

Tedeschi R.G., & Calhoun, L.G. (1996). The posttraumatic growth inventory: Measuring the positive legacy of trauma. *Journal of Traumatic Stress, 9*(3), 455–471.

Tierney, A.L. & Nelson, III, C.A. (2009). Brain development and the role of experience in the early years. *Zero Three, 30*(2), 9–13.

Totton, N. (2015). *Embodied relating: The ground of psychotherapy.* Routledge.

Tryon, G.S. & Winograd, G. (2011). Goal consensus and collaboration. *Psychotherapy, 48*(1), 50–57.

Vuorre, M., Orben, A. & Przybylski A.K. (2021). There is no evidence that associations between adolescents' digital technology engagement and mental health problems have increased. *Clinical Psychological Science, 9*(5). https://doi.org/10.1177/2167702621994549

Wallin, D.J. (2007). *Attachment in psychotherapy*. Guilford Press.

Wampold, B.E. (2015). How important are the common factors in psychotherapy? An update. *World Psychiatry, 14*(3), 270–277.

Wampold, B.E., Baldwin, S.A., Holtforth, M.G. & Imel, Z.E. (2017). What characterizes effective therapists? In L.G. Castonguay & C.E. Hill (Eds.), *How and why are some therapists better than others? Understanding therapist effects* (pp.37–53). American Psychological Association.

Wampold, B.E. & Brown, G.S.J. (2005). Estimating variability in outcomes attributable to therapists: a naturalistic study of outcomes in managed care. *Journal of Consulting and Clinical Psychology, 73*(5), 914–923.

Wampold, B.E. & Imel, Z.E. (2015). *The great psychotherapy debate: The evidence for what makes psychotherapy work* (2nd ed.). Routledge.

Watson, J. (Ed.). (2019). *Drop the disorder! Challenging the culture of psychiatric diagnosis.* PCCS Books.

Wiebe, S.A. & Johnson, S.M. (2016). A review of the research in emotionally focused therapy for couples. (2016). *Family Process, 55*(3), 390–407.

Wilkinson, R. & Pickett, K. (2009). *The spirit level: Why equality is good for everyone.* Penguin Books.

Wilkinson, R. & Pickett, K. (2018). *The inner level: How more equal societies reduce stress, restore sanity and improve everyone's well-being.* Allen Lane.

Williams, S. & Paisner D. (2009). *On the line.* Grand Central Publishing.

Wolitzky-Taylor, K.B., Horowitz, J.D., Mark B., Powers, M.B. & Telch, M.J. (2008). Psychological approaches in the treatment of specific phobias: A meta-analysis. *Clinical Psychology Review, 28*(6), 1021–1037.

World Health Organization. (2022, June 8). *Mental disorders.* [Online.] https://www.who.int/news-room/fact-sheets/detail/mental-disorders

Worley-James, S. (2022). *Online counselling: An essential guide.* PCCS Books.

Xavier, A. (2020). The big issue: Playing the numbers game. *Therapy Today, 30*(6). https://www.bacp.co.uk/bacp-journals/therapy-today/2020/july-2020/playing-the-numbers-game/

Zeng, N., Pope, Z., Lee, J.E. & Gao, Z. (2018). Virtual reality exercise for anxiety and depression: A preliminary review of current research in an emerging field. *Journal of Clinical Medicine, 7*(3), 42.

Name index

J

K

L

M

N

O

X

Z

Subject index

S

V

W

PCCS Books

Also in the *Straight Talking Introductions* series

A Straight Talking Introduction to the Power Threat Meaning Framework: An alternative to psychiatric diagnosis

Mary Boyle and Lucy Johnstone

A Straight Talking Introduction to Psychiatric Drugs: The truth about how they work and how to come off them

Joanna Moncrieff

A Straight Talking Introduction to Psychiatric Diagnosis

Lucy Johnstone

A Straight Talking Introduction to the Causes of Mental Health Problems

John Read and Pete Sanders

A Straight Talking Introduction to Children's Mental Health Problems

Sami Timimi

A Straight Talking Introduction to Emotional Wellbeing: From mental illness to Mad Studies

Peter Beresford